MASTERING THE INNER GAME OF WEIGHT LOSS

An Easy-to-Follow Guide to Permanent Weight Loss Without Going on a Diet

Mastering the Inner Game of Weight Loss: An Easy-to-Follow Guide to Permanent Weight Loss Without Going on a Diet

Copyright © 2017 by Ellen G. Goldman

All Rights Reserved

Published by EllenG Coaching, LLC, 2018

No part of this publication may be reproduced, distributed, or transmitted in any form or by any means, including photocopying, recording, or other electronic or mechanical methods, without the prior written permission of the publisher, except in the case of brief quotations embodied in critical reviews and certain other noncommercial uses permitted by copyright law.

Cover and Interior Design by Misha Gericke

DISCLAIMER

While I am a Certified Professional Wellness Coach and a Certified Personal Trainer, I am NOT a physician or registered dietician. This guidebook is NOT intended as medical advice, exercise prescription, or to replace the recommendations of your personal physician or any other health care provider.

As with any new program you may undertake, it is advisable to discuss your plans to improve your diet and increase your activity level with your physician before you begin. This is especially important if you are under a doctor's care for a medical condition or taking prescribed medications. Get the clearance from your doctor, share the information in this guidebook, and then get started!

If you have any questions or concerns, I am available through my website, www.EllenGCoaching.com or by email at ellen@ellengcoaching.com.

Ellen G. Goldman, M.Ed., NBC-HWC

National Board Certified Health & Wellness Coach

MASTERING THE INNER GAME OF WEIGHT LOSS

An Easy-to-Follow Guide to Permanent Weight Loss Without Going on a Diet

ELLEN G. GOLDMAN

CONTENTS

Copyright Page and Disclaimer
2

Title Page
3

Contents
5

Dedication
15

Introduction
17

Tip #1: Eat often and eat light—never go more than four hours without a meal or snack.
23

Tip #2: Eat within one hour of awakening.
28

Tip #3: Eat the last meal or snack of the day at least three hours before bedtime.
34

Tip #4: Combine protein, complex carbohydrates, and a small amount of healthy fats at every meal and snack.
39

Tip #5: Always carry portable healthy snacks when away from home for long stretches of time.
46

Tip #6: Preplan meals and snacks into your day every morning when reviewing your schedule.
51

Tip #7: Rate your hunger on a scale from one to five before you eat anything, with one being ravenous and five being stuffed.
56

Tip #8: Eat slowly and mindfully. Stop when satiated, not stuffed.
62

Tip #9: Taste a small amount of desserts and treats; savor and enjoy them, then put the fork down.
67

Tip #10: Eat food high in fiber every day.
73

Tip #11: Eat at least five servings of fruit and/or vegetables daily.
79

Tip #12: Be mindful; check in with yourself before making food choices.
86

Tip #13: Eat a large salad or bowl of soup before entrées.
91

Tip #14: Avoid buffets. They are an invitation to overeat.
96

Tip #15: Don't ignore hunger.
103

Tip #16: Don't head to the supermarket hungry. Eat a healthy meal or snack before buying groceries.
108

Tip #17: Read food labels.
114

Tip #18: Avoid buying trigger foods that you know will cause you to lose control and overeat. Keep them out of your home and office.
121

Tip #19: Drink water before meals.
127

Tip #20: Drink lots of clear liquids all day—primarily water, seltzer, or tea.
133

Tip #21: Weigh in at least once a week. Ignorance is not bliss when it comes to weight loss.
138

Tip #22: Have a happy target weight to strive for, with a five-pound acceptable weight range.
144

Tip #23: Strength train at least twice a week for a minimum of 20 minutes.
151

Tip #24: Do 30 minutes of aerobic exercise at least five days each week.
158

Tip #25: When short on time, squeeze in a quick workout rather than not at all. A little exercise is always better than no exercise.
165

Tip #26: Schedule exercise into your calendar in advance and treat it like a business appointment. Non-negotiable!
171

Tip #27: Join a group exercise class that is fun and that you will look forward to. If it's gratifying, there's a good chance you will go.
178

Tip #28: Exercise with a buddy—a friend or family member. Commitment to exercise increases when you partner up.
184

Tip #29: Tag exercise with another activity you enjoy: listening to music, reading, watching TV, or walking with your dog.
189

Tip #30: Increase daily movement whenever possible.
194

Tip #31: Wear a pedometer every day.
202

Tip #32: Check serving sizes on foods' labels. Do the math in order to keep portion sizes and consumption in line with your weight loss goals.
208

Tip #33: Use measuring cups and spoons as serving utensils.
215

Tip #34: Do not serve family style, except when it comes to salads, veggies, or fresh fruit.
220

Tip #35: Get seven to eight hours of sleep every night.
227

Tip #36: Wear form-fitting clothing.
234

Tip #37: Cook healthy foods in advance and freeze in individual containers.
240

Tip #38: Avoid multitasking while eating. That means no eating in front of the TV, or while talking on the phone.
246

Tip #39: When socializing, focus on the people, not the food.
252

Tip #40: Paint your kitchen and dining room, and buy plates and utensils in soft hues such as blue, green, or gray.
260

Tip #41: Designate the kitchen as a room to be used only for food prep and eating.
266

Tip #42: Replace oversized plates, bowls, and glasses with smaller ones.
274

Tip #43: Keep healthy foods in clear containers and bowls, on counters and at eye level in the fridge.
281

Tip #44: Keep treats and temptations in opaque containers situated in the back of the refrigerator, freezer, or cabinets.
289

Tip #45: Use positive self-talk, mantras, and visual reminders of your goals.
296

Tip #46: Ask those you love and trust for the support and encouragement you need in order to succeed in your weight loss efforts.
305

Tips #47–#50: Mint, mint, mint, and more mint. Use mint to boost your weight reduction efforts: inhale, ingest, brush, and chew.
316

Tip #51: Experiment with yoga or meditation.
323

Tip #52: Respect your intuition and listen to your body.
330

Note from the Author
337

Acknowledgments
339

About the Author
341

Appendix A
343

Appendix B
346

Appendix C
351

Appendix D
354

DEDICATION

This book is dedicated to all of my current, past, and future clients. I learn as much from you as I hope you learn from me. Thank you for your willingness to kick dieting and embrace a new approach to managing your weight, and for your leap of faith in allowing me to guide you through my beliefs and methodologies.

This book is also dedicated to my amazing mom, Laura Greene, who tried a zillion different diets, finally chucked them all, and indeed became a master at the inner game of weight loss.

INTRODUCTION

Welcome to Mastering the Inner Game of Weight Loss: An Easy-to-Follow Guide to Permanent Weight Loss Without Going on a Diet!

I'm delighted that you have purchased a copy of this guidebook. It is the accumulation of years of working with clients to achieve sustained weight loss. Every successful individual came to the realization that success is not achieved by going on a diet, but rather by changing his or her mind, attitude, and approach to weight loss. Those who achieve sustained weight loss do so by slowly shifting or eliminating old, sabotaging habits and creating new, healthy ones that easily fit into their lifestyle—regardless of how hectic and complicated that lifestyle might be.

After more than 30 years in the health and fitness industry, I know for sure that, although some individuals will lose *some* pounds by following a specific diet plan, most people *do not* achieve *permanent* weight loss by going on diets.

Success is achieved when you change the way you think about eating, your relationship with food, and your daily lifestyle habits. Not just habits concerning the food you eat and your daily movement, but also patterns related to stress management, sleep, your environment, and even the folks you spend time with. This guidebook will present 52 highly effective ways to reshape your thoughts, habits, and environment to build a lifestyle that will support losing the excess pounds you have been carrying and help you keep them off for good!

You are about to be introduced to many small, manageable steps that can begin to add up to massive change. But first...

Let me give you a brief idea of who I am and why I am so passionate about helping you achieve sustained weight loss without reverting to rigorous diet and exercise plans— which I believe is doomed to fail you in the long run.

My choice of a career in health and wellness was shaped by the experiences I had growing up—although I didn't realize it at the time—with a Mom who was *always* dieting. Mom was constantly "on" or "off" her diet. She was either working hard to take off some pounds before some big family event or an upcoming summer vacation, or because her doctor was concerned about her blood pressure or cholesterol.

Being told that taking off weight would improve her health profile, along with the desire to look and feel better, kept mom motivated. Mom's struggles were not because she didn't try or didn't want to lose the weight badly enough.

Her days were often marked as "good" or "bad," dependent on her ability to resist the forbidden foods, and her closet was filled with a multitude of sizes, which marked her up-and-down journey in the battle to lose weight.

I can vividly remember her going off to Weight Watchers meetings, trying the newest diet recommended by her girlfriend who had recently lost weight, or buying the foods listed in the Take Off 10 Pounds Fast article from Women's Home Journal. Whether it was the Atkins Diet, the Grapefruit Diet, or Pritikin Plan, each promised the ever-elusive prize: a lower number on the scale and a smaller clothing size. It was exhausting to watch, and surely more exhausting to live that way.

Not much has changed since those days. Although some of the diets are still around, some have faded from view, and others keep appearing. Dieting remains as popular, and more so now than ever. As a matter of fact, it is estimated that at any given time, 70 percent of adult females and 30 percent of adult males are on a diet. And whether it's the newest fad diet, a medically supervised program, or the promise of a new pill, supplement, or drink, people will try almost anything in their obsessive desire to lose weight.

The sad part is, as mentioned earlier, although many diets will result in some weight loss in the short term, few people achieve what they are really looking for—permanent weight loss, resulting in a body in which they feel comfortable, healthy, and happy.

At some point in my young adult years, I remember watching Mom and thinking to myself, "There has got to be a better way! There is absolutely no way I am going to live my life going on and off diets."

So I went off to study, learn, and practice what the science and research concerning health and wellness was teaching us. Maintaining a healthy body weight and living a life of energy and vibrancy is the result of daily habits—habits concerning not just food consumption, but movement, stress management, sleep patterns, the environment surrounding us, the support and relationship we have with others and, most importantly, our mindset. In other words, our daily thoughts and actions will determine the shape of the body we live in—not choosing to follow one diet or another.

That is what this guidebook will help you do; to develop those habits and teach you how to determine what works best for you and your unique lifestyle and situation. So let's dive in and show you how to make the best use of this guidebook.

Although there are 52 tips—no coincidence that there are 52 weeks in a year—you should go at your own pace. However, I suggest you focus on one tip each week. Experiment with the idea, practice, and repeat. Internalize the lessons. Take a little time to go through the questions, reflections, action steps, and exercises at the end of each tip. If at the completion of the week, you feel ready to embark on a new tip, move on. Just don't stop practicing the tip from the previous week.

If, however, you feel you need more time on one, and are not ready to build in the next, that's OK! There's no urgency or deadline you must meet. We are working on changing old habits, and creating new ones. And that takes time. However, once you've ingrained these habits into your lifestyle, they will just become a part of who you are and how you live. More than that, they *will continue to support you in losing the excess weight and keep it off for good*!

Also, feel free to jump around. You don't have to follow these guidelines one after another. Although they tend to build on each other, some will feel more enticing to you than others. By all means, start with the tips that excite and interest you. You might even feel that some of the ideas presented aren't relevant for your situation—and that's just fine. The important thing is that you stay open to trying new ideas, be patient with yourself, and have fun! This approach is not about starvation or deprivation, failure or success, being "good" or "bad." It's about creating a lifestyle you can live with, feel comfortable with, *and* that will finally help you to achieve permanent weight loss without having gone on a diet.

So dive in and begin your journey into *Mastering the Inner Game of Weight Loss*. If you ever need some extra support or assistance along the way, don't hesitate to reach out to me. Even if you just want to share your success! I would love to hear from you and how this guidebook is helping you achieve your wellness goals.

By the way, Mom did eventually lose the weight. At the time of this publishing, she is 96 years old! She no longer beats herself up daily because of the number on the scale. Mom enjoys eating delicious, healthy fare, and occasionally indulges in decadent desserts and treats. Walking, water aerobics, dancing, and living a busy, connected social life have all contributed to her longevity.

Although I may have started my journey looking to escape the lifestyle Mom had, now I admire her tenacity and am inspired on a daily basis to follow her lead. I hope you will be too!

TIP #1

Eat often and eat light—never go more than four hours without a meal or snack.

I am excited to begin this adventure with you. With each brief but thorough explanation of how to easily tweak one lifestyle habit at a time, you will master the inner game of weight loss. By integrating one tip a week for the next 52, you will not only take off excess pounds but begin to feel more energized, focused and productive. Without further ado, let's dive into Tip #1.

Eat often and eat light means never going more than four hours without a healthy meal or snack. This idea just might be the most important tip I'll share, and changing this one habit can dramatically enhance your entire weight loss journey.

If you have been struggling to lose weight, "eat often and eat light" might seem counterproductive to achieving your goal. Shouldn't you be eating less and trying to eat less often? Most individuals who attempt to slim down think that the longer they wait before eating or snacking, the better the outcome will be. But the truth is that our bodies need a steady source of fuel to function and feel good. That fuel comes from the foods that we eat and liquids that we drink. By maintaining a regular intake, our blood sugar remains even.

Why is this important? Because it is a stable level of blood sugar that helps keep our brains performing well cognitively (or, in simpler terms, thinking straight). When blood sugar dips, we become cranky, irritable, and irrational, not to mention hungry! If we deprive ourselves of nutrients for an extended period, through a complex physiological system, our brilliant bodies will produce a hormone that screams, "Feed me! Feed me!" And that's when we reach for any edibles we can get our hands on. Usually, those are not nourishing, good-for-you foods. Instead, they are simple carbohydrates loaded with sugar, such as cookies, candy bars, or fast food items. Those types of foods digest quickly and provide the instant boost in energy we need.

The problem is that we'll inevitably come crashing down just as quickly, which, in turn, sends us right back to the vending machine, refrigerator, or junk food cabinet—whichever one we can gain access to first! So, if weight loss and feeling good is your goal, you want to avoid this blood sugar roller coaster. You can do that by eating often and eating light.

Understand that there is nothing magical about the four-hour time frame. It takes approximately one hour to digest 100 calories. For your last meal to sustain you about four hours, it should be an acceptable size that leaves you satisfied, rather than stuffed; probably around 400 calories. Eat less, and you'll likely become hungry sooner—perhaps three hours after your meal. Consume a healthy mix of complex carbohydrates like fruit, vegetables, or grains; some lean protein such as eggs, poultry, meat, fish, or legumes; and a little healthy fat. That's the kind of meal that will keep you feeling satisfied until it is the appropriate time to eat again. The trick is when you begin to feel hungry—truly physically hungry—to take note, stop what you are doing, and eat. If it's the appropriate hour for a full meal, then take the time to eat it. If not, find (or have on hand) a healthy, 100–200-calorie snack to bridge the gap until your next meal.

So there you have an essential tip to commence this week: **Never skip meals; do not go any more than four hours without eating; and choose light, healthy, and satisfying fare.** By gradually incorporating this pointer and those that follow, you will create positive inroads on your weight loss journey. You are on your way toward new habits and a lifestyle that perpetuates sustainable weight loss and well-being!

FOOD FOR THOUGHT... QUESTIONS & REFLECTIONS

1. What parts of the day are you most vulnerable to going long stretches (more than four hours) between meals?

   _____

   _____

   _____

2. What changes can you make in your behaviors and habits that will ensure that you eat light and healthy at least every four hours?

   1. _____

   2. _____

   3. _____

   4. _____

ACTION STEPS & EXERCISES

1. Using the form provided in Appendix B, or any notebook or smartphone app you prefer, keep a simple food journal this week. Include the time you eat, the foods and drinks you consume, and

a *brief* description of how you feel before and after eating.

2. If skipping meals or going long stretches without food is the norm for you, set an alert on your computer or smartphone to remind you to stop and eat meals and snacks at appropriate times throughout your day.

3. This week, when you notice physical sensations of hunger, take note of how many hours it has been since your last meal or snack. At the end of the week, ask yourself what you have learned or noticed since doing so.

TIP #2

Eat within one hour of awakening.

This tip will focus on breakfast. The word literally means the meal that "breaks the fast." Breakfast provides the body and the brain with fuel after a night of having abstained from eating. Let's face it: During sleep, your body doesn't require much fuel. However, once you are up and active, you need energy to function optimally. Without breakfast, you're effectively running on empty.

Start your day off on the wrong foot, and there's a good chance that the rest of the day might not run as smoothly as you would prefer. Minus the necessary brain fuel, you lack the ability to think as clearly or perform at your best, which can lead to feelings of stress, overwhelm, and fatigue. The result: you often reach for comfort foods that are high in calories and low in nutritional value. If you haven't eaten a healthy breakfast, it's harder to ignore the cream doughnuts in the company break room or your own kitchen.

Consuming a healthy breakfast has been linked to numerous health benefits. It provides you with energy to start a new day and helps with weight control and improved performance throughout the day, no matter what you are trying to achieve. Beginning the day with a well-balanced meal that supplies adequate protein, carbohydrates, and fiber keeps hunger at bay and allows you to make wise decisions regarding the meals that follow. Some examples of a nutritious breakfast include half of a whole grain English muffin spread with lite Swiss cheese, and topped with a poached egg, or oatmeal with fresh fruit and a sprinkle of nuts.

While it might seem that you can save calories by skipping breakfast, this does not prove an effective strategy for weight reduction. Many studies, in both adults and children, indicate that breakfast eaters tend to weigh less than those who forgo breakfast. Breakfast skippers tend to eat more at the next meal, or they nibble on high-calorie snacks to stave off hunger. The National Weight Control Registry is an organization whose members have all lost at least 30 pounds and maintained that weight loss for at least one year. Approximately 80 percent of Registry members regularly eat breakfast. Also, a study from Loyola University found that eating within one hour of awakening can boost one's metabolism by up to 20 percent for the remainder of the day.

Even when I explain to clients the many benefits of

eating within one hour of awakening, a common challenge I often hear is, "I'm just not hungry in the morning. The thought of eating makes me feel sick." If this describes you, you likely feel that way for one of two reasons: First, there's a very good possibility that you are simply not in the *habit* of eating breakfast. Your body has learned not to expect food in the morning, so ghrelin, the hormone that gives us the message we are hungry, is suppressed. Or, second, perhaps you overate, ate too late, or both, the previous night.

In either case, know that you can retrain the body to desire fuel in the morning. First and foremost, you must master the mindset that eating within one hour of awakening is good for your waistline and your life! Recognize that eating too much and too late is negatively impacting your health and weight, and work on modifying that habit.

You can start small. Begin with something light, such as a banana, a cheese stick, or even a cup of juice. As eating a bit in the morning becomes more tolerable, gradually add a little more food during your new meal time. Before you know it, you'll wake feeling hungry and begin craving a healthy breakfast.

Ready to give this tip a try? Start implementing the morning ritual of **eating within one hour of awakening**. You will also begin enjoying a new kind of day—fresh, alert, raring to go, and *mastering the inner game of weight loss*!

FOOD FOR THOUGHT... QUESTIONS & REFLECTIONS

1. At what time do you usually wake up?

   _____

   At what time do you usually eat breakfast?

   _____

2. What constitutes your typical breakfast?

   _____

   _____

3. If you typically skip breakfast, what are some of your reasons for doing so?

   _____

   _____

   _____

4. What behaviors could you alter to ensure that you eat a healthy breakfast within one hour of awakening?

   A. Habit tweaks the night before:

      i. _____

ii. _____

B. Habit tweaks in the morning:

i. _____

ii. _____

EXERCISES & ACTIONS STEPS

1. This week, keep track in the breakfast section of the Food Journal (see Appendix B), or add to your Food Journal from last week's tip, the time you awake each morning, the time you eat breakfast, and the foods and drinks you consume.

2. Write down what you notice in terms of how you feel, both physically and emotionally, on the days you eat breakfast, compared to days when you skip eating within one hour of awakening.

_____
_____
_____
_____
_____

TIP #3

Eat the last meal or snack of the day at least three hours before bedtime.

There seems to be an ongoing debate and conflicting information as to whether or not late-night calorie intake triggers weight gain or inhibits weight loss. I am aware that many individuals would argue that there is not enough research to support the belief that consuming the bulk of calories late at night definitively leads to weight gain.

Studies addressing whether eating later in the day

impacts weight gain consider groups of individuals who take in a similar number of calories and types of food each day, and then manipulate when those calories are consumed. If you are eating a reasonably healthy diet, and remaining within a calorie range that makes sense for your body type and activity level, the time that you eat does not seem to make a big difference regarding weight reduction.

However, in the real world, outside of the research lab, excess late-night calories are not exclusively attributable to eating a late dinner. Rather, they result from snacking on too many unnecessary calories while watching TV, picking at leftovers when cleaning up after supper, or eating to help keep yourself alert when you're burning the midnight oil.

So, if you were to set this rule in place—no eating within three hours of bedtime—a significant portion of extra calories would be eliminated daily. And that could easily bring about some weight loss without changing anything else in your diet or exercise plan.

Another reason to consume the majority of calories earlier in the day is simply that you do not require much fuel while asleep. Therefore, it's preferable to shift your routine and ingest the greater share of your calories during the daytime when you need the energy that you obtain from food to perform all of your daily activities. To me, that certainly makes sense.

Keep in mind that a three-hour window allows the body to fully digest the food from the last meal or snack so that you don't go to bed on a full stomach, which can cause digestive issues and interfere with your sleep. Also, eating too late at night often results in waking the next morning without feeling hungry. That, in turn, leads to skipping breakfast, the unfavorable results of which we addressed previously in Tip #2.

Nevertheless, on occasion, you might find yourself up later than usual, and whether due to a very light dinner, or no dinner at all, you find yourself feeling physically hungry before bedtime. In those instances, a light snack is acceptable. You don't want hunger to keep you awake or disturb an otherwise good night's sleep. When that occurs, a cup of chamomile tea with some graham crackers; a mug of hot chocolate made with skim milk; a banana; or even a small bowl of cereal all constitute good choices. They will take the hunger pangs away, allowing you to drift off and sleep soundly through the night.

The takeaway for Tip #3 is that if you are a late-night eater, it can serve you well to **adjust your nighttime habits and eat the last meal or snack of the day at least three hours before bedtime**. Hopefully, this week's tip will guide you in making another transition to ultimately help you reach your weight loss goal.

FOOD FOR THOUGHT...
QUESTIONS & REFLECTIONS

1. On average, at what time to you go to sleep?

   _____

2. On a typical night, at what time do eat your last meal/snack?

   _____

3. What behaviors can you modify to ensure that you eat/snack earlier in the evening, and stop eating at least three hours before bedtime?

   _____

   _____

   _____

   _____

ACTION STEPS & EXERCISES

1. This week, add to your food journal from the past couple of weeks the time you consume your last meal or snack each day, what you consume, and the time you go to bed.

2. Take notice of how you feel, both physically and emotionally, and your quality of sleep on the nights you stop eating at least three hours before going to bed as compared to evenings when you continue to eat until bedtime.

_____

_____

_____

_____

_____

_____

_____

TIP #4

Combine protein, complex carbohydrates, and a small amount of healthy fats at every meal and snack.

There are three sources of food: carbohydrates, proteins, and fats. Combining all three at every meal and snack is not only important for weight loss and maintenance, but also for overall health and performance.

Allow me to provide a brief and simplified nutrition

lesson to make sure you understand the differences between each food source, and the role each plays in providing fuel for your body.

Carbohydrates are divided into two categories—simple and complex. Sugar, white bread, white rice, chips, baked goods, and most junk foods are primarily made up of simple carbs. They have little nutritional value and only add unnecessary calories to your diet. Complex carbs—foods such as whole grains, brown rice, quinoa, oatmeal, and all fruits and vegetables—are the body's primary sources of energy and offer rich supplies of fiber. In addition, they help regulate blood sugar levels. The more active you are and the more you exercise, the more your body needs carbohydrates to supply your muscles with the energy essential to functioning.

High-quality proteins contain the amino acids that are the basic building blocks of muscle as well as the many enzymes, hormones, neurotransmitters, and antibodies that our bodies require. Protein also supports metabolism and helps stabilize our energy levels by way of its effects on insulin and blood sugar, plus it keeps us satisfied. We want to acquire protein from lean meats, poultry, fish, legumes, nuts, eggs, and low-fat dairy products.

Last but not least, we need fat in our diets. Fat is NOT the enemy. Essential fats provide vital nutrients that do a variety of good things for our body. Dietary fats are crucial to physical growth, cognitive development, and cellular processes. They assist with the performance of our nerves and brains. Fat helps maintain healthy skin and hair and is needed for transporting the fat-soluble vitamins A, D, E, and K throughout our bloodstreams. And fat is what makes so many of our foods taste good!

The tricky part is that not all fats are created equal,

and fats are very dense sources of energy. Whereas every gram of carbohydrate or protein supplies the body with four calories, every gram of fat supplies the body with nine calories. So choose wisely. A little fat goes a long way in adding flavor and satiation along with its health benefits. We want to minimize saturated fats and eliminate trans fats completely. Yet we can enjoy nourishing fats, such as those found in vegetable oils; fresh fish like salmon, halibut, and albacore tuna; avocados; nuts; and many dark green leafy vegetables, like spinach.

Do understand that most foods we eat already contain a combination of at least two, if not all three, of these food sources. For instance, cheese contains both protein and fat. Spinach has both carbohydrates and fat. Each source—carbohydrate, protein, and fat—offers its own combination of nutrients, vitamins, and minerals to keep the body functioning optimally. So combining each at every meal and snack ensures that you will get all of the vitamins and minerals you need.

Additionally, each food source varies in terms of the amount of time it takes for energy release and digestion. When you eat a carbohydrate alone, you will get a quick burst of energy, but it will be followed soon after by a crash. Add some protein and fat, and just as the energy from the carbohydrate is depleted, digestion of the other food sources begins. Therefore, you end up feeling satisfied for a much longer period. And the more satisfied you feel after meals and snacks, the less you will reach for excess, non-nutritious calories.

So rather than just an apple, eat an apple with a tablespoon of peanut butter. Add cut fruit and a handful of nuts to a container of low-fat yogurt in the afternoon, and you won't be hungry again until dinnertime.

There you have it: **Combine all three food sources—protein, complex carbohydrates, and fats—during each meal and snack,** and you will enjoy all of the unique health benefits each has to offer. Your blood sugar will remain steady, keeping your moods and energy levels stable, and you will also feel satisfied.

FOOD FOR THOUGHT... QUESTIONS & REFLECTIONS

1. Browse through the food journals you have kept the last few weeks, or write down in the space provided below the typical foods you choose throughout the day. Identify the food sources of the items that make up your typical meals and snacks.

    1. Breakfast

    _____

    _____

    _____

    2. Lunch

    _____

    _____

    _____

    3. Dinner

    _____

    _____

    _____

4. Snacks

_____

_____

_____

2. What do you need to **add** to your current diet (meals and snacks) to create the ideal combination of healthy carbs, proteins, and fats?

_____

_____

_____

_____

3. What do you need to **eliminate** from your current diet (meals and snacks) to create the ideal combination of healthy carbs, proteins, and fats?

_____

_____

_____

_____

ACTION STEPS & EXERCISES

1. At least once a week, stock up on an array of proteins, complex carbohydrates, and healthy fats for the entire household.

2. Plan each meal in advance to include all three food sources.

3. Rid your home of non-nutritive or flat-out unhealthy foodstuffs from each food source category.

TIP #5

Always carry portable healthy snacks when away from home for long stretches of time.

Losing weight doesn't have to mean elaborate, time-consuming diet and exercise plans. This week's tip is one that can have a significant impact and influence on your weight loss efforts, and it is so easy to implement: **Always have healthy, portable snacks accessible when you're away from home for long stretches**

of time.

Why is this so significant? Think back to the very first tip: Eat often and eat light—never go more than four hours without fuel. I hope that by now you are thinking of food and the calories you consume as your fuel—the energy that keeps you going throughout the busy day and keeps your brain alert and sharp so that you can make wise decisions.

You might ask, "Why are you encouraging me to eat snacks when I am trying to lose weight?" Because when it comes to weight loss and healthy living, hunger and fatigue are your enemies. Going too long without proper fuel will leave you both excessively hungry and fatigued. It will also lead to choosing high calorie, high-fat foods between meals, unless you have a healthy snack accessible within easy reach.

If you aren't in the habit of carrying nutritious snacks with you, you will find yourself hungry and tired without healthy options all too often. Then the only choice might be reaching for vending machine junk food in the middle of the afternoon. Or you'll be eating the candy in the checkout line at the market or grabbing a bag of chips at the gas station convenience store. Therefore, to avoid being caught off guard, be prepared with wholesome snacks. Exchange those impulsive food choices with healthy fuel, and you will reduce your intake of excess, non-nutritious calories.

Let's consider the easiest way to apply this strategy. First, you will need to have nutritious snacks in your home to take with you when you leave. The next time you are at the grocer's, stock up on apples, cheese sticks, nuts, and protein bars. These are just a few examples of healthy edibles that are easy to bring with you when you leave home. Don't forget a water bottle too. Dehydration can mask itself as either hunger or fatigue, or both.

Second, while reviewing your daily calendar, mentally walk through your day in regard to when and what you will be consuming. If you eat breakfast at 7:00 a.m. and plan on traveling to a meeting mid-morning, but not joining your friend for lunch until 1:30 p.m., you are going to need a healthy snack in between. Are hours spent in an airport going to be part of your day? Don't be left at the mercy of poor, non-nutritive choices at the airport kiosks. In case you don't know this, although you cannot bring liquids, you *can* carry food through security checkpoints. If you regularly have business meetings that run late on Wednesdays, causing you to eat dinner later than usual, fuel yourself beforehand with a healthy snack. When driving straight from the office to the supermarket, nibble on a healthy snack before you head out the door. Remember, however, that you can't do that unless you have it with you.

In short, review the day's schedule each morning (or the night before). **Plan ahead and pack nutritious snacks to bridge extended hours between meals.** Then watch your energy soar and your waistline shrink.

FOOD FOR THOUGHT... QUESTIONS & REFLECTIONS

1. Which parts of your typical day lend themselves to long hours between meals?

   _____

   _____

   _____

2. What foods do you already have in your home that will make for good snacks to take with you when you go out?

   _____

   _____

   _____

3. What foods will you add to your shopping list to serve as portable, healthy snacks?

   _____

   _____

   _____

   _____

ACTION STEPS & EXERCISES

1. If you don't already have one, purchase or download a calendar or daily planner. (See Appendix C for suggestions.)

2. Choose a consistent time to review your upcoming day, either the night before or early in the morning. If you will be on the road or away from home for any significant stretch of time, pack some healthy snacks into your bag or briefcase.

3. Make sure to include wholesome snack foods on your shopping list.

TIP #6

Preplan meals and snacks into your day every morning when reviewing your schedule.

Today's tip is a bit of an extension of last week's. We addressed why it is essential to include healthy snacks in your day to bridge the hunger gap between meals, and how, if you don't have them with you, chances are you will opt for high-calorie, non-nutritious foods instead.

This week, we'll go one step further in planning, and that is to begin thinking about your meals as well. All of this is leading up to becoming *proactive*, *rather than reactive*, to your body's need for food. The goal is to avoid being stuck without healthy food available when it is time for a meal. Without preplanning, there is a good chance you'll find your only alternative is high-calorie, unhealthy fare. Or even worse, you'll end up in a circumstance where you're so hungry that you just don't care and then reach for anything you can get your hands on, as long as it is fast and convenient. When those types of situations become less frequent, and that behavior is no longer part of your daily habits, the pounds start melting off.

Taking a few minutes every morning to plan can make a huge difference, not only in the number on the scale, but also in your energy levels, your productivity, and your overall health. Just as you started to practice packing and bringing snacks with you on days you are away from home for long stretches of time, now you can begin to look at the bigger picture.

For most, breakfast is not a big issue when eaten at home. If you stocked your kitchen properly, you have plenty of healthy choices. But what about the days when you have a breakfast meeting? I used to go to a monthly breakfast meeting during which they only served bagels and pastries. Those do not support my health and weight maintenance goals. So on those days, I would always pack my yogurt and fruit and bring them along. You may be thinking that seems embarrassing or a bit obsessive. Nevertheless, my health is far more important to me than what others think—and truthfully, many people would say, "Gosh, I wish I thought to do that. You're so smart." I'm not necessarily smart. I'm simply a good planner.

Next, let's consider lunch. Will you be home or on the road? Do you need to brown bag it today? If yes, take a couple of minutes to do so. It doesn't require much time to pack a turkey sandwich, apple, and water bottle into a bag. Or, if you have a lunch date, make sure it is at a restaurant you know has menu choices that will reinforce your weight loss efforts.

Do you know what you'll be preparing for dinner? Make sure to remove anything you might need from the freezer to defrost. Otherwise, you may end up picking up a pizza on the way home.

I think you understand where I am going with this. When it comes to weight loss and maintenance, *failure to plan is planning to fail*. Planning is an easy habit to develop, but it takes time and practice. So I challenge you this week. **Spend a few minutes when reviewing your schedule every morning or evening before to preplan meals and snacks into your day.**

FOOD FOR THOUGHT... QUESTIONS & REFLECTIONS

1. Do you review your schedule every day? If not, when would be a consistent daily time when you could begin doing so?

   _____

2. What has been your experience with preplanning meals and snacks? If you aren't in the habit of doing so, what are your thoughts about making this part of your daily or weekly routine?

   _____

   _____

   _____

   _____

   _____

   _____

   _____

   _____

3. What behaviors could you adjust in the mornings or evenings to ensure that you plan daily meals and snacks?

    _____

    _____

    _____

    _____

ACTION STEPS & EXERCISES

1. Google "Meal and Snack Planners" online (either as an App, downloadable form, or pre-printed pads). Choose one that appeals to you and order it. Once it arrives, experiment with planning out a week's worth of meals and snacks. Most planners will allow you to create your grocery list based on your choices.

2. Block out time in your week that is convenient for you to preplan on a regular basis.

3. Each morning (or the evening before, if you prefer), check your meal planner along with your day's schedule. Transfer any frozen foods you may need for dinner to the refrigerator, and pack your lunch and snacks if you will be away from home.

TIP #7

Rate your hunger on a scale from one to five before you eat anything, with one being ravenous and five being stuffed.

Now, here is a tip that may ruffle your feathers: Rate your hunger on a scale from one to five before you eat anything, with one being ravenous and five being stuffed. I can imagine you thinking, "Ellen, you've got to be kidding me. You expect me to stop every time I'm about to eat something and rate my hunger on a scale of one to five? That's crazy." Well, bear with me as you read further. While I assure you that this is not something you will need to practice for the rest of your life, I will explain why it is an excellent exercise for you to try for a week or two.

The problem I'm addressing is that we seldom recognize real, physical hunger. We are surrounded by food and eat so often that we lose track of when the body is presenting real signs of hunger. Usually, the first time we recognize these signals is when we have already gone too long without eating and end up with one ravenous sensation. Does this ring true for you?

Your aim should be to eat when you are at about a three on the scale, which is when you first notice signs of hunger. Perhaps your stomach is growling, and you may feel a slight decrease in your energy level or concentration and an empty feeling in your belly. Once you have partaken in a meal or snack, aim to stop at a four rating; when you are satisfied, rather than at a five, when you're stuffed (you know, that post-Thanksgiving-Dinner feeling).

These days, we are constantly surrounded by food. We eat all the time and rarely is it because we recognize that we are genuinely, physically hungry. *When the clock says 6:00 p.m., it must be time for dinner. When you hear and smell the popcorn popping in the movie theater, you want some and eat some regardless of the fact that you might have just had a meal. When you see the doughnuts in the cafeteria, you help yourself to one.*

What if, instead, you were to briefly pause right before grabbing a tempting bite, take a breath, and ask yourself, "What am I feeling now on the hunger scale?" One=ravenous. Two=very hungry. Three=hungry. Four=satisfied. ("I'm not in need of food," or, "I've had enough.") Five=stuffed. ("I've eaten recently and am still full. There is no need for more food.)

The goal for weight loss—and all-around good health—is to be aware of your body's hunger signs, and respond as soon as you hit that three on the hunger scale. This idea brings us all the way back to Tip #1; eat often and eat light. Remind yourself that, if you only eat when you are hungry—not because you see the food; smell the food; or are bored, procrastinating, or not paying attention—you will cut out an enormous amount of excess calories from your daily intake. Eliminating those calories over the course of one week, two weeks, or a month can add up to a fair number of pounds disappearing.

So here is my challenge for you, not for the rest of your life, but just for one week (or two): When you notice that you are about to reach for food, simply pause for a moment. Take a breath. Then ask yourself that question: "How hungry am I on a scale of one to five?" By all means, if you find yourself at one, two, or three, go ahead and eat. If the answer is four or five, walk away. If you did hit that one or two, remember to pay attention the next time you hear that growling, grumbling sound coming from your stomach or your intuition saying, "Hmm, I think I'm hungry." Then stop what you are doing and either eat a meal if it's the appropriate time, or munch on a snack to bridge the gap before your next meal.

By simply becoming aware, you can take the time to rate your hunger and then choose whether or not to eat at a given moment. Once you practice this exercise for a week or two, you will become more attuned to your body's genuine signs of hunger. Learning to listen to your body and make better decisions will promote healthy eating and enhance your weight loss efforts.

FOOD FOR THOUGHT... QUESTIONS & REFLECTIONS

1. How often do you eat for reasons other than hunger?

   _____

2. How do you feel physically after eating most meals?

   _____

   _____

3. How often do you feel stuffed (a rating of five) after eating?

   _____

   What circumstances or environmental situations might contribute to overeating?

   _____

   _____

4. What signs or sensations do you notice when you begin to realize you are hungry?

   _____

   _____

5. What signs or sensations do you notice when you have overeaten?

ACTION STEPS & EXERCISES

1. This week, each time you are ready to reach for food, rate your hunger.

2. If you determine that you are at an appropriate level of hunger and you partake in a meal or snack, rate your hunger again when you're done eating.

3. Be mindful. Pay attention to the physical signs of hunger.

4. Practice this exercise for one to two weeks. How has using the Hunger Scale impacted on your journey towards healthy eating and weight loss?

TIP #8

Eat slowly and mindfully. Stop when satiated, not stuffed.

I will now share a tip that is remarkably simple to incorporate and so effective that, if you changed nothing else, over time you might just shave off a few extra pounds just by following this advice. That's not to say I want you to ignore the other tips and tricks you have integrated over the past few weeks, or to stop any other efforts you have been employing to lose excess weight, but rather that you add this one to your toolbox. Because according to research, if you practice slow and mindful eating, you will consume fewer calories. After all, the total number of calories you eat, compared to the total your body needs to meet daily demands, will determine whether you lose, gain, or remain at the same weight.

My recommendation, backed by science, is to **eat slowly and mindfully, and to stop when satiated, not stuffed**. Numerous studies have shown that when we eat more slowly, we take in fewer calories. Several researchers have proven that when we increase the number of times we chew before swallowing food, there is a reduction in the total number of calories consumed. Interestingly, individuals who maintain a healthy weight tend to eat much more slowly than people who are overweight.

Taking your time helps you to avoid overeating. When you eat too quickly, your body doesn't have enough of an opportunity to undergo its natural appetite-signaling process or proper digestion. There is a complex physiological and hormonal link that occurs between the time we put food into our mouths, chew, and swallow, to the time it travels to the stomach to digest. We know it takes approximately 20 minutes before the signal arrives at the brain and tells us that we've had enough. When we rush through our meals or snacks, by the time we receive that message, there is a good chance we have overindulged and can end up feeling stuffed, rather than satisfied. Add the element of mindfulness to slowing down; that means carefully paying attention to the taste, texture, smell, and overall enjoyment of what we are ingesting. Mindful eating not only helps us to eat less, but also to enjoy our food more and feel emotionally satisfied as well as physically satiated.

As you begin experimenting with these habits, here are several helpful hints: Make a decision that you will not multitask while eating. If you are going to take the time to eat, treat it as a welcome break from the busyness of your day. Stop and take a breath. Tell yourself to relax and enjoy. Then savor the foods you are eating. Deliberately slow down your chewing. Put down your sandwich or fork in between bites. Take a few sips of water in between as well—this is also an excellent way to increase your water consumption! Then, when you have finished about three quarters of what's on your plate, pause and take a few minutes to relax. Ask yourself, "Am I satisfied?" If the answer is "Yes," then push your plate away.

Adjusting your eating routine further should augment your weight reduction efforts. If you find it easier, you can even break down Tip #8 and **focus on eating more slowly first**. Once that feels habitual, become more deliberate and attentive as you begin the practice of mindful eating.

FOOD FOR THOUGHT... QUESTIONS & REFLECTIONS

1. How would you describe the rate at which you consume most meals and snacks?

   _____

   _____

   _____

2. How might you adjust your behaviors and environment to help implement the practices of slower and mindful eating on an ongoing basis?

   _____

   _____

   _____

   _____

   _____

   _____

   _____

   _____

ACTION STEPS & EXERCISES

1. Keep track of the time it takes you to eat each meal and snack.

2. Stop eating when there is still a small amount of food left on your plate.

3. Make a conscious effort to take note of when you feel satisfied vs stuffed. Use the Hunger Scale presented in Tip #7.

4. Purchase or download a book or CD that guides you through the practice of mindful eating. Check out the resources listed in Appendix A.

TIP #9

Taste a small amount of desserts and treats; savor and enjoy them, then put the fork down.

I know you'll love Tip #9! Yes, I *am* suggesting that you taste a small amount of desserts and treats; savor them, enjoy them, and then *put the fork down*.

Your immediate response to this advice might be, "What? Ellen, you're telling me to enjoy desserts and treats when I'm trying to lose weight? Have you lost your mind?" And my answer would be, "I have not lost my mind and, although this tip seems illogical, you will read here why it makes so much sense." I have been a Wellness and Weight Loss Coach long enough to have learned that you are setting yourself up for failure by adhering to the hard-and-fast rule to eliminate desserts and treats from your diet.

The ideal approach to weight reduction and maintenance doesn't include deprivation because deprivation eventually leads to lack of control. When you make an absolute decision to forego desserts and treats, you might be able to stick with that plan for about a week; maybe a month; or even a couple of months. Willpower may work for the short term. After all, you feel like you have the fortitude and are highly motivated to lose weight.

However, when you consistently say, "No, no, no!" to something you want, sooner or later, you will crash. And when you do give in to the temptation, you will ultimately get carried away. Rather than just a small taste, you will find yourself eating the whole enchilada and looking for more.

It is much, much healthier to make some proactive decisions beforehand in respect to desserts and treats. Let's say that you have a special celebration to attend—a birthday or anniversary—and there will be a delicious cake at the event. Or perhaps you are going to your favorite restaurant that serves the most incredible tiramisu dessert, which you've enjoyed in the past. Relying on your willpower may just not be enough to resist those temptations.

Instead of sacrificing such goodies altogether, a better approach is to say to yourself, "I am going to enjoy a taste of that dessert guilt-free, and I'm going to balance the excess intake by cutting back somewhere else." Perhaps skip the bread before dinner or have one glass of wine that night instead of two.

So when that special treat arrives at the table, have a taste. When you take that mouthful, really savor it. Be mindful of the sensation; how delicious those one or two bites are. Next, put the fork down, push the plate away, and consider yourself finished with that meal. Hopefully, you already decided on one dessert for everyone to share, and your companions will be enjoying their tastes as well.

I would love for you to try this strategy even if it feels a bit risky. I can imagine some people's response to this challenge: "No way! If I have one small bit, I'm not going to be able to control myself." If this sounds like you, that assertion is probably the story you have been telling yourself for a while. And that kind of mindset needs to be adjusted. Begin by repeating, **"I can control myself. I can have one small taste, enjoy it guilt-free, and put my fork down."** Practice that mantra, and what is likely a novel approach for you, and see the positive impact it has when it comes to indulging a bit *and* losing weight.

FOOD FOR THOUGHT... QUESTIONS & REFLECTIONS

1. What are the typical thoughts that run through your mind when confronted with a high-calorie and/or high-fat tasty treat or dessert?

   _____
   _____
   _____
   _____
   _____

2. What is your common behavior when in a situation where a decadent dessert or snack is readily available, if not sitting right in front of you?

   _____
   _____
   _____
   _____
   _____

3. When you make a decision to lose weight, do you usually decide certain foods are totally "off limits"? If yes, which foods do you try to eliminate from your diet?

_____

_____

_____

_____

_____

4. When you know that you will be in a situation tempted by unhealthy treats, what might you do to set yourself up for success?

_____

_____

_____

_____

_____

ACTION STEPS & EXERCISES

1. Obliterate the "no desserts or treats" rule.

2. Begin to change your mindset. Repeat the "I can control myself..." mantra as above, especially before you are face-to-face with a delicious dessert or similar treat.

3. When you do take those one or two mouthfuls, remember to focus on and savor the taste and accompanying sensations.

TIP #10

Eat food high in fiber every day.

This week, we're going to review tip #10: **Eat foods that are high in fiber every day.** Now, I'm sure you're aware of all the information available regarding the many health benefits of eating more fiber. I think it's important that you not only understand what fiber is and what foods to consume to increase your intake, but also why.

Dietary fiber is found mainly in fruits, vegetables, whole grains, and legumes. It is typically classified as either soluble, meaning it dissolves in water, or insoluble, meaning it does not dissolve in water.

Soluble fiber is found in oats, peas, beans, apples, citrus fruits, carrots, barley, and psyllium. Studies show soluble fibers can help lower blood cholesterol and glucose levels.

Insoluble fiber is found in complex carbohydrate foods such as whole wheat flour, wheat bran, nuts, beans, and many vegetables, like cauliflower, broccoli, Brussels sprouts, and green beans, to name a few. Even potatoes can be good sources of insoluble fiber. This type of fiber is involved in helping your digestive system work properly and increasing your stool bulk. That is why it helps prevent or relieve constipation.

Because dietary fiber includes the parts of plant foods that your body cannot digest or absorb, it passes relatively intact through your stomach, small intestine, and colon and out of your body. Some refer to this as the *scrub brush effect*—meaning that fibers help to clean out bacteria and other buildup in your intestines. There is evidence that diets high in fiber can reduce the risk of colon cancer. A healthy diet that includes soluble fiber may also reduce the risk of developing type 2 diabetes.

Certainly, there are enough health benefits to justify increasing your daily intake of fiber. Add to those the positive effect it has on weight loss and I'm sure I now have your attention. Because fiber slows the rate at which sugar is absorbed into the bloodstream, it keeps your blood sugar levels from spiking too fast. Consequently, you avoid the crash and burn often felt after eating simple carbohydrates—foods high in sugar or white flours. We know that crash and burn leaves you feeling hungry too soon and can, therefore, lead to overeating.

High-fiber foods generally require more time to chew, which slows down eating and gives your body time to register that you're no longer hungry—that you've had enough. And because these foods are so filling, especially when coupled with protein and some healthy fats, you stay full longer. Most importantly, high-fiber diets tend to be less "energy dense," meaning they provide fewer calories for the same volume of food.

When you increase your intake of high-fiber foods, you have less room for junk food. Speaking of which, please don't be fooled by the manufacturing companies that are jumping on the bandwagon and adding processed fibers such as inulin, polydextrose, and modified starches. Most processed fibers do not do as much good as intact, unprocessed fiber. And since the health agencies claim that most consumers' diets are fiber deficient, smart manufacturers are increasing the appeal of purchasing foods that scream, "High in fiber!" Adding processed fibers does not turn cookies, brownies, snack bars, and shakes into healthy foods, and those certainly won't help your weight loss efforts.

So how should you increase the amount of fiber you consume daily? Here are a few suggestions:

- Eat, rather than drink, your fruits and vegetables. Choose an orange instead of orange juice, or tomatoes and carrots in place of vegetable juice.

- Include vegetables—preferably fiber-rich types like greens and broccoli—as part of every meal and snack. Aim for the higher end of the recommended 5–9 servings per day.

- Keep the edible peels on fruits and

veggies. That's where you'll get the highest concentration of fiber.

- Eat more beans, lentils, and split peas. Order hearty bean and vegetable, broth-based soups.

- Consume oatmeal or high-fiber, low sugar cereals for breakfast.

- Whenever possible, replace white foods such as bread, pasta, and rice with brown, whole-wheat, or whole-grain options.

- Snack on nuts, berries, and air-popped popcorn.

Among the many benefits of fiber-rich foods are those that advance your endeavors to reduce weight. Therefore, on the journey of sustained weight loss (and overall health enhancement), it behooves you to **modify your existing habits to integrate fare that is high in fiber**. Begin this week to create a new behavior that becomes a regular part of every day.

FOOD FOR THOUGHT... QUESTIONS & REFLECTIONS

1. What high-fiber foods do you regularly consume?

   _____

   _____

   _____

   _____

2. What low-fiber, high-calorie, sugar-rich foods might you consider eliminating from your diet, and what might you replace them with?

   _____

   _____

   _____

   _____

ACTION STEPS & EXERCISES

1. Research comprehensive lists of fiber-rich edibles so you can add more variety to your diet.

2. Research simple recipes that center on or include foods that are high in fiber.

3. Include on your shopping list fiber-rich foods that you want to incorporate into your meals and snacks, along with those needed for new recipes you want to try.

TIP #11

Eat at least five servings of fruit and/or vegetables daily.

It's likely you've heard it before. Every health organization out there touts the benefit of eating a minimum of five servings of fruits and vegetables a day. This advice is for good reason, because fresh fruits and vegetables are nutrient-packed. They supply our bodies with so many of the vitamins and minerals we need to function well and stay healthy. Folate, iron, magnesium, potassium, and Vitamins A and C are just some of the many nutrients found in the vast variety of plant food available to us. A diet high in produce may reduce the risk of many diseases, including cardiovascular disease and some cancers. Produce is high in fiber, which is so essential for heart and digestive health.

But have you wondered why increasing your intake of veggies and fruits is so important when it comes to weight loss? Why is it that a diet high in produce is one of the secret weapons for taking off excess pounds and maintaining a healthy weight?

Fruits and vegetables are referred to as nutrient-dense foods. That means you can eat a lot for fewer calories. And that is very significant in terms of keeping you feeling satisfied when you are trying to cut back on your total caloric consumption (which, after all, is the key to losing weight). You can eat a large volume of produce, which fills you up and keeps your desire for food in check.

When you are filling up on nutrient-dense foods, you leave little room for nutrient-empty foods such as cookies, chips, or candy. Those choices are high in calories, but low in, or have no, nutritional value. Not where you want to bank your calorie intake for good health and weight loss!

Fruits and veggies are also quick and easy eats. They don't require a lot of preparation, are highly portable, can be eaten on the road, and are available in many different forms. Although I always prefer fresh produce, frozen, canned, or dried are good, viable options in a pinch, all still high in health benefits and low in calories for high-volume consumption.

The extensive variety of produce available keeps eating interesting. Often, clients complain to me that they get so bored of the "healthy foods" they are consuming when they are trying to lose weight. If you can relate, it's time to widen your horizon. There is a myriad of choices and ways to prepare vegetables and fruits. You must simply be willing to try something new and experiment with new recipes. I'm sure you've heard the advice that, to reap all of the health benefits, you should eat the rainbow. It is easy to do with all of the choices available, and that will definitely keep you from getting bored.

Right now, my favorite kitchen tool is called a Veggetti. I use it to make spaghetti-like strands from zucchini or squash. Prepared just the way I might make traditional pasta—with either tomato sauce, pesto, garlic and oil, and topped with turkey meatballs—these vegetable strands create a delicious meal. It's very filling and contains much fewer calories than if I used spaghetti or noodles.

If I've convinced you that increasing your consumption of fruits and vegetables can help you on your weight loss journey, and you are ready to commit to doing so, here are some quick ideas on how to easily incorporate them into your daily diet:

- Make veggie omelets for breakfast.

- Add sliced cucumber, tomato, and arugula to sandwiches.

- Keep bags of baby carrots or sugar snap peas on hand to munch on while cooking or driving long distances.

- Make fruit smoothies for a quick breakfast or midday pick-me-up.

- Try frozen grapes for a refreshing snack.

- Eat oven-baked sweet potato fries.

- Toss in leftover veggies with chicken or steak strips for a quick stir-fry dinner.

The list goes on and on. Use your imagination and creativity.

But, of course, it all begins with having these healthy fruits and vegetables on hand, in sight, and available. Next time you head to the grocery store, stock up on produce and keep those items in open containers on your table or in the fridge. Don't hide them away in drawers where you'll forget them. Out of sight, out of mind. In sight, in your mouth.

Today, **begin thinking about which fruits and vegetables you can include in your diet plan, rather than which foods to eliminate**. Perhaps you can commit to trying one new vegetable or fruit a week. You'll soon see how easy it is to include at least five servings in your daily consumption.

FOOD FOR THOUGHT... QUESTIONS & REFLECTIONS

1. Which fruits and vegetables do you regularly include in your daily diet?

   _____

   _____

   _____

   _____

   _____

   _____

2. What is the average number of servings of produce you currently eat per day?

   _____

3. List ideas you have on how to increase your daily servings of fruits and vegetables.

   _____

   _____

   _____

4. Which new varieties of fruits and vegetables are you willing to try?

ACTION STEPS & EXERCISES

1. This week, commit to trying one or two new fruits or vegetables which you haven't tasted in the past. Either add them to your shopping list OR, once at the supermarket or farmer's market, choose what looks appealing to you.

2. Find one new vegetarian recipe that you are willing to try. Plan on your calendar when you will

grocery shop for any items you need and when you will cook this dish. This can be a main course, side dish or even a healthy dessert. Be creative and have fun!

3. Using some of the ideas you came up with above, begin adding more fruits and/or vegetables to the meals you commonly eat.

TIP #12

Be mindful; check in with yourself before making food choices.

Let's delve into this week's tip: **Be mindful; check in with yourself before making food choices.** Ask yourself if you're physically hungry or eating for another reason, such a boredom or procrastination. If the answer is "No, I am not really hungry," walk away and find another activity to occupy your time.

It sounds so straightforward and logical—common sense. However, common sense doesn't always mean common practice. Obviously, if we stopped eating for emotional reasons and only ate for nourishment—that is, when we are physically hungry—we would take in much fewer calories per day.

What, when, and how much we eat is often automatic—done with little or no thought. We pass through the kitchen, see the open cookie jar, and grab one. In a restaurant, we eat everything on our plates just because the food is in front of us. We're bored and can't make up our minds as to what we want to do next, so we find ourselves munching away while staring out of the window. All of this adds up to hundreds of excess calories consumed per day. Over time, those extra calories lead to extra pounds gained.

Imagine what might happen if you consciously decide to press the pause button before reaching for food every single time you are about to eat? What if you were to stop, take a breath, and ask, "Am I hungry? Truly physically hungry?" Note the time. When was your last meal or snack? Is your stomach growling, feeling empty? If the answer is no, you have a decision to make—walk away. You must learn to resist eating when it's not related to physical hunger, especially if you're trying to lose weight or concerned about maintaining your current weight.

Perhaps you can ask yourself, "What is it that I need?" Maybe it's a break from work. Your brain is tired. Your body is achy from sitting at the computer, or you just feel depleted. Food will probably not satisfy that need the way a brief walk, stepping outside for some air, or even a chat with a coworker will. If you are angry, stuffing yourself will only make you more upset—this time at yourself. It's better to deal with your anger in a constructive manner. Talk to a friend or battle it out with your loved one. In other words, do something that will relieve and resolve the anger. Are you bored? Prepare a list of projects you've intended to do and start one. Dive in and get started on that work project you've been thinking about. Read that novel on your nightstand. Clean that closet that's overflowing. Call that friend you've been missing.

Learning to be mindful of "why" you are eating takes practice. You have to make a conscious decision that you will pause before making all food choices. Start with a one-day commitment to do so, and see what happens. You might even jot down or journal about what you notice and learn about your habits. Awareness, as we say, is always the first step in changing our behaviors. Just being aware of how often you reach for food when you aren't hungry will help you cut back on the frequency of doing so.

This week, **begin to weave in mindful practice regarding when you eat.** You just might see the number on the scale start to drop. And you might end up feeling more productive too.

FOOD FOR THOUGHT... QUESTIONS & REFLECTIONS

1. How often do you pause and think about when and what to eat before reaching for food?

   _____

   _____

2. Reflect on your most common triggers (emotional and environmental) for eating when you do so for reasons other than physical hunger. What strategies might help you avoid eating when those circumstances occur?

   _____

   _____

   _____

   _____

   _____

   _____

   _____

   _____

3. What might you do to remind yourself to stop and think before eating? (Example: Put a post-it note on the refrigerator that says, "Are you hungry?")

_____

_____

_____

_____

ACTION STEPS & EXERCISES

1. Consider keeping a journal for a few days. Note each time you eat and what your motivation is in that instance. (This may be difficult in certain situations, such as in the workplace. During those times, be sure to take mental note as to why you are making the food choices that you are.)

2. Make a list of the activities or projects you might work on to distract yourself from eating when you are not physically hungry, and keep it in a visible place. Refer to it the next time you notice you are reaching for food but not because of physical hunger.

TIP #13

Eat a large salad or bowl of soup before entrées.

One of the nutritional tools I use to help myself and clients eat healthily and balance caloric intake is to eat a large bowl of salad or a non-cream-based soup before lunch or dinner.

Eating a salad or veggie soup before your meal does more than help you meet your daily vegetable quota. Starting your meals this way may be an effective strategy in helping you decrease your total calorie consumption during lunch or dinner, which, in turn, can help you manage your weight.

Non-cream-based soups and salads share a common denominator: they are both nutritionally dense—meaning high in nutrients with relatively few calories. There is also a high water content in both, which keeps you hydrated and feeling full. Hearty salads and vegetable and bean soups increase fiber and add staying power. So not only will you fill up with fewer calories, but you'll also stay satisfied longer.

However, you must watch your portions and avoid high-calorie salads full of too many extras like bacon, croutons, cheese, dried fruit, or cream-based dressings. The same goes for soups. Onion soup is great but not when made with a huge chunk of bread in the middle and the crock covered in melted gruyere cheese.

I find this tip especially useful in restaurants. Since the average restaurant entrée consists of significantly more food and calories than a meal we eat at home, starting a restaurant meal with a salad or soup has many advantages. It takes the edge off your hunger, slows the time you spend at the table and gives you the chance to recognize you are full before devouring everything on your plate. Then you can pack up half of your entrée and you've got a gourmet lunch for the next day.

At home, this can be a great tool as well. Spend a little time on weekends chopping vegetables so you can easily combine them to create salads. Use some of those vegetables to cook up large batches of soups. They are easy to make, freeze beautifully, and can be available quickly at the end of the work day. Soups and salads are easily portable and make great first courses before lunch at the office or dinner at home. With enough healthy vegetables and some added protein like lean chicken, turkey, beans, or tofu, you can turn them into a meal.

In one study, researchers found that people who begin their meals with a simple vegetable soup eat about 20 percent fewer calories than those who don't. It didn't matter if the soups are chunky or pureed, as long as they were low in total fat and calories.

Eating a large portion of "low-calorie" salad before the main entrée proved to be another effective approach to cutting calories. This method increased fullness while decreasing the total caloric intake of the meal by 12 percent.

If those percentages sound a bit small and you think they won't make that much of a difference, imagine cutting back 12 to 20 percent of total calories at several meals a week for an entire month. If you go ahead and implement this week's tip, you just may notice the numbers on the scale moving in the downward direction without having gone on a diet!

FOOD FOR THOUGHT...
QUESTIONS & REFLECTIONS

1. What type of appetizers do you typically consume before a main entrée?

   _____

   _____

2. How often do you order soup or salad at restaurants?

   _____

3. What type of soups do you usually eat?

   _____

   _____

4. What kinds of dressings and toppings do you add to your salads?

   _____

   _____

   _____

5. If you typically consume high-calorie appetizers, calorie-laden soups and salad dressings, what ideas do you have for consuming healthier choices?

_____

_____

_____

_____

_____

ACTION STEPS & EXERCISES

1. Research recipes for healthy vegetable and protein-laden soups. Stock up on the ingredients and cook soups, beginning with one recipe at a time, until you learn to make a variety of non-cream-based, nutritious, and filling concoctions.

2. Prepare batches of soups to be served with lunches and dinners that will last you and your family for days.

3. Purchase only nutrient-rich salad ingredients, plus low-calorie, low-sugar dressings. Use dressing sprays for a lighter touch. Or eliminate packaged dressings and dribble a healthy oil (e.g. olive oil or avocado oil) and balsamic or red wine vinegar over your salad. Go even lighter with a splash of lemon or try it with no dressing at all.

TIP #14

Avoid buffets.
They are an invitation to overeat.

My kids grew up learning what they now call "Mom's mantras." There were several sayings which I hope conveyed important messages about how to live happily and healthily in the world.

When it came to "Mom's mantras" on eating, there is one I have often heard them repeat to their friends: **"Buffets are an invitation to overeat."**

How I came to that conclusion was based on intuition alone. I noticed early on that, whenever I was at a buffet, I left feeling stuffed, uncomfortable, and annoyed with myself for overeating. I grew to hate that feeling. Despite how good the food may (or may not) have tasted, every time I ate at a buffet, I overate.

Little did I know back then that research substantiates this theory. Brian Wansink, one of the premier researchers in the area of Mindless Eating (and, by the way, the author of the book with the same title) proved in the research lab that the more choices we have, the more calories we consume.

Increasing the variety of food available increases how much we eat. This behavior results from what is called "sensory-specific satiety," fancy words that mean our senses become numbed if they continually experience the same stimulus. Sensory-specific satiety affects our taste buds. The first bite of anything is almost always the best. The second, a little less, and the third, less again. At some point, we get tired of the chocolate cake. But if we can then switch to the strawberry shortcake or the apple pie, our taste buds are excited and happy again. So we change to a new food choice and eat some more.

This tendency to overeat when offered greater variety holds true even when eating healthy foods. Dr. Barbara Rolls and her team at Penn State showed that if people were offered an assortment of three different flavors of yogurt, they were likely to consume an average of 23 percent more than if they had been offered only one flavor.

If you're trying to control your weight, one obvious tool is to avoid buffets as much as possible. That may mean speaking up for yourself when choosing a restaurant with friends and family. Most hotels offer more than one restaurant choice. When traveling, make sure you choose the à la carte restaurant rather than the buffet or the eatery that serves family style.

However, there will be times when you have no choice. Either you are at a catered event that is serving buffet-style or perhaps a family gathering where dinner is presented that way. I only serve buffet-style for holiday dinners at my home. With guest lists that can range between 20 and 30 people, I can't possibly prepare a seated, plated dinner.

But don't despair. There are several tips you can use when faced with the buffet and trying to watch your weight. First, remember that awareness is half the battle. Remind yourself in advance that buffets are tempting and easy opportunities to overindulge. So, first and foremost, don't show up starving. Have a small, healthy snack an hour or so before the event. Don't skip meals beforehand thinking you'll "save up" your calories for the buffet. That will usually result in you consuming more once you get there. When you arrive, peruse the entire table first before making any choices. Then choose foods you love or are unique from what you normally can get. Do not waste your calories on humdrum items just because they are in front of you.

Start with some salad or non-cream-based soup, if offered. (Recall Tip #13?) Another smart strategy is to never have more than two items on your plate at a time. You can go back if you are still hungry, but the lack of variety slows you down, giving you a chance to digest and feel satiated. Try to stand or seat yourself away from the actual buffet table, so it's out of sight while you eat. Remember, most of the time when challenged by a buffet, you're at a social event. Try to focus on the people, not the food. Engage in conversation and social connection. After all, it's not polite to talk with your mouth full.

So, to sum up Tip #14, **avoid buffets whenever possible but, if faced with one, approach the situation with a clever plan in mind.**

FOOD FOR THOUGHT... QUESTIONS & REFLECTIONS

1. How often, and in which situations, do you find yourself in the presence of buffet-style eating?

   _____

   _____

   _____

   _____

2. Reflect on your experiences when faced with a buffet. On a scale of 1–10, with 1=ravenous and 10=Thanksgiving-dinner-food coma, how do you usually feel when you leave that event?

   _____

3. What events do you have coming up where there will be a buffet table?

   _____

   _____

   _____

   _____

4. What strategies are you willing to try to avoid overeating when faced with buffet-style meals?

_____
_____
_____
_____
_____
_____

ACTION STEPS & EXERCISES

1. Be cognizant whenever you know that an event will serve buffet-style. Think in advance about how you will handle your eating behavior.

2. Have a healthy snack about an hour before a buffet-style event.

3. Once at a buffet, enlist the many suggestions below to ensure you don't succumb to the typical pattern of overeating:

    a. Think before you choose the foods you will put on your plate.

    b. Take only two items at a time.

c. Start with a healthy salad or soup, if available.

d. Choose special foods that you particularly like and don't get to eat often.

e. Situate yourself as far as possible from the buffet table.

f. Focus on socializing, rather than eating.

TIP #15

Don't ignore hunger.

As soon as you recognize the physical signs of hunger (growling stomach, slight light-headedness, focus and energy draining), stop and eat a nourishing snack or, if it's the appropriate time, have a meal. Letting yourself get too hungry leads to poor choices and overindulging.

Are you one of those folks who get so busy during the day that you ignore the signs of hunger, figuring you don't have time to stop to eat and actually think that's a good thing because you're trying to lose weight? Do you feel that skipping meals is an excellent way to save calories? Do you believe that being famished is par for the course if you are on a diet?

If so, you're in good company. Lots of people think that, in order to lose weight, they have to accept they'll have lots of hunger pangs throughout the day and that feeling deprived is just part of the equation. *You don't have to* experience constant hunger to lose weight and, as a matter of fact, you shouldn't have to. In my experience, hunger is the enemy when it comes to losing weight, and ignoring your hunger will set you up for failure.

If you're always hungry, you are not eating enough. Not consuming enough food can trigger a breakdown of calorie-burning muscle, slow down your metabolism, and even compromise your immune system. Undereating starves the lean tissue you need to nourish your body and can cause ravenous hunger that leads to bingeing.

So many people go on low-calorie diets, thinking they'll be able to foster the willpower to ignore or tolerate hunger. And they may succeed for a couple of days, or perhaps even a couple of weeks. But constant hunger and feelings of deprivation usually lead to crashing and caving in. It's hard to make reasonable, healthy choices when you're depriving your brain and body of necessary fuel.

The vicious cycle of deprivation followed by over-consumption leaves you feeling bad about yourself and defeated. Perhaps you give up, go back to the habits you had before the diet and maintain them until the next time you muster enough motivation to try again. So let's give up the myth that low- or very-low-calorie diets and skipping meals are the road to permanent weight loss success. Let's get sensible and realize that the key to success is nourishing your body properly throughout the day.

That begins with recognizing the signs of hunger and responding immediately. Mild to moderate hunger is your body's way of telling you it needs more fuel. A healthy, balanced meal should leave you feeling full and energized for three to four hours. Then your hunger should return, which is a signal that it is time to refuel.

Rather than going on a diet, begin to plan for three healthy meals a day and one or two snacks. It will take experimenting with your intake and timing of eating so that you will begin to feel appropriately hungry at mealtimes and satisfied, not stuffed, after eating. You'll also need to pay attention to which foods keep you satiated and provide the most staying power for the lowest caloric intake. You'll feel full a lot longer after having a breakfast of scrambled eggs and a whole grain English muffin instead of a doughnut and coffee.

Remember when incorporating this week's tip that small steps lead to huge results. So, **once you're aware that you are physically hungry, pause and eat a nutritious snack or meal.** Keep in mind that hunger is counterproductive to making wise decisions when it comes to eating properly. Now you understand why.

FOOD FOR THOUGHT... QUESTIONS & REFLECTIONS

1. How do you feel when you recognize you're physically hungry? What messages does your body give you?

   _____

   _____

   _____

   _____

   _____

   _____

2. What is your typical response when you realize you're feeling hungry? Is your instinct to ignore hunger, or to stop what you are doing and get something to eat?

   _____

   _____

3. Does your daily schedule allow for consistent break times for meals and snacks when hunger sets in, or does it fluctuate? How might you make

adjustments so you can include a healthy snack or meal when you become hungry?

_____

_____

_____

_____

_____

_____

ACTION STEPS & EXERCISES

1. This week, be mindful— increase your awareness of the signs of physical hunger. Stop as soon as reasonably possible to have a snack or meal. Note any changes you notice regarding your moods, energy levels, and ability to resist unhealthy fare.

2. Do not go more than four hours without a snack or meal.

3. Experiment with your dietary intake to determine how much food will satisfy but not over-stuff you.

TIP #16

Don't head to the supermarket hungry. Eat a healthy meal or snack before buying groceries.

It's pretty obvious that, if you want to lose weight, you need to eat nutritiously. That means having healthy groceries on hand. But one of the most frequent problems I encounter with those struggling to manage their weight is a lack of forethought to their meals.

Have you ever found yourself standing in front of the fridge with the door open, staring and wondering, "What should I eat for lunch or cook for dinner?" Is your answer any of the following: "Whatever is in the house," "There's always takeout," or "I'll get in the car and head to the nearest diner or deli, or take a frantic trip to the supermarket"?

If so, you're making your weight loss journey more difficult, if not impossible.

Not having nutritious, enjoyable foods accessible in your home is stressful, time-consuming, expensive, and often leads to eating high-calorie, non-nutritious foods that don't support weight loss. How much better would it be to have a fridge and pantry filled with nutritious and delicious choices all the time? However, to make that happen, you will need to routinely think about what foods you want in your home, make a list, and then take the time to go to the grocery store.

But don't go to the supermarket when you're hungry! Trying to shop while your stomach is growling leads to impulse buys and emotionally charged choices rather than rationally thought out ones. You may even find yourself munching on a candy bar while in the checkout line.

Be proactive rather than reactive.

Think about your week. We're all different, and what works for me may not work for you. I know that the best time for me to shop is on a Tuesday late afternoon, after my last appointment of the day. Mondays are lousy grocery shopping days in my town; the shelves are empty and the produce looks tired, droopy, and picked-over after the busy weekend crowds. New deliveries arrive on Tuesday mornings. When I go at around 5:00 p.m., the store is relatively empty. And this works for me because, truth be told, I really don't enjoy supermarket shopping. If the store is crowded, I like it even less. But I *do* enjoy having healthy food in my home.

So I arrive with a list in hand of everything I'll need for the upcoming week's meals. I use the weekend to plan my menu. A quick stop towards the end of the week to fill in fresh produce keeps me to no more than two visits to the market per week. Shopping from a list, I can get in and out quickly and, since I already know what I'm preparing for that night (I keep Tuesday suppers quick and easy), dinner is on the table on time.

Now it's your turn. What would be the best way for you to keep your home stocked with healthy fare? The choices are many: scheduled supermarket shopping, grocery delivery services, meal-prep subscription plans. However, whichever you choose, there will be times you need to head to the food stores. So be prepared.

And don't head to the supermarket hungry. Take a few minutes to eat a nutritious snack before going grocery shopping.

For me, 5:00 p.m. is several hours past lunch. If I haven't had my afternoon snack, that's way too many hours to keep my hunger in check when faced with all the supermarket temptations. By now, you know that a combination of complex carbs, protein, and a small amount of healthy fat is what you want to include in all of your meals and snacks to keep your blood sugar even and hunger at bay.

Yogurt and fruit, hummus and carrot sticks, and a fruit smoothie made with almond milk are a few snack ideas for before you go shopping. If all else fails and you are pressed for time, eating a high-quality protein bar while driving to the market will work as well. Stay away from high-sugar, salty, or fatty snacks—they'll make you crave more of the same and, as you know, the grocery store is filled with those kinds of foodstuffs.

So there you have it. To lose or maintain a healthy weight, **plan your meals in advance, shop from a list, schedule specific times to go to the supermarket, and always go right after a meal or a healthy snack.**

FOOD FOR THOUGHT... QUESTIONS & REFLECTIONS

1. What system do you have in place to plan out your meals for the week and create a shopping list? If you don't have one, how might you tackle this challenge in a way that will fit into your lifestyle? What systems could you put in place and what would support your being successful?

   _____
   _____
   _____
   _____
   _____
   _____
   _____

2. Think about your typical week. What would be the best times for you to go food shopping—both when it's convenient for you and also when there are the freshest and healthiest choices available?

   _____
   _____

ACTION STEPS & EXERCISES

1. Create a detailed shopping list to include the healthy foods you like to have on hand and ingredients needed to make meals for the week.

2. Schedule the day and time you plan to shop on your calendar.

3. Choose a healthy snack to eat before heading to the market, if it will be more than three to four hours since you have last eaten.

TIP #17

Read food labels.

Whether you're trying to lose weight or just eat healthier, reading nutrition labels is an excellent habit to develop. It can be quite helpful for making wise choices when purchasing food. There is a wealth of information available on food labels, but unfortunately, you'll probably find it quite confusing unless you're a registered dietician. It's time-consuming too.

It would take a significant amount of text to explain all that is found on labels. Here I hope to give you a few guidelines and shortcuts on what, in my opinion, is the most relevant when weight reduction is your goal. If you want to stock your fridge and pantry with foods that will support your weight loss efforts, you'll need to pay some attention to those food labels.

When attempting to lose weight, the instinct is only to check total calories and make food selections based solely on that information. However, making a choice based on calories alone, without paying attention to serving size, can be a huge mistake! Let me give you an example: You want a protein bar to eat after your workouts. Calorie count reads 150. Good choice, right? Wrong. If you look at the serving size, it says half a bar. That will cost you 300 calories. You could end up ingesting the same amount of calories you just expended exercising. Or perhaps your favorite breakfast cereal lists 110 calories per serving. So you happily munch on it each morning. Upon closer look, you see the serving size says one-quarter of a cup, and you consume closer to a cup each day. Mistakes like those leave you wondering why you aren't losing weight since you're eating such healthy foods. Therefore, you must consider calories and serving size together and do the math.

Moving on down the label, check the total fat content. Healthy fat is an essential ingredient for staying well and keeping you satisfied. It also makes food taste good. But it's relatively high in calories for each gram: 9 calories per gram vs 4 calories per gram in carbs and protein. So a little goes a long way. I try and keep my fat calories to about 30–35 percent of my total calories each day. Yours might be different, depending on your genetics, body composition, health profile, etc. But my rule of thumb is to stay away from foods in which there are more than 3 grams of fat per 100 calories. And I prefer that fat to be attained primarily from unsaturated rather than saturated or trans fat.

You already know I advocate high fiber and low sugar as an overall guideline for healthy eating and weight loss. So check the fiber and sugar contents next. A useful criterion is to look for at least 3 grams of fiber per serving in any product that contains grains, including bread, crackers, pasta, and even some soups. In general, the higher the fiber and the lower the sugar, the healthier the product is for you.

Looking at the sugar content can be confusing. This number doesn't always distinguish between naturally occurring sugars (like lactose in milk or fructose in fruit) and added sugar (like high-fructose corn syrup or brown rice syrup). A better move is to look at the ingredient list for sources of *added* sugar. Look for the words sugar, as in palm sugar or invert sugar; sweetener, as in corn sweetener; or syrup, as in brown rice syrup or malt syrup. Also watch for words ending in "-ose," like fructose or glucose. If sugar is one of the first few ingredients listed, put that item back on the shelf. Ingredients are listed by volume, in descending order. So the further down the list the sugar appears, the better.

Salt is a tricky one. Most health organizations say we should limit our daily intake to 2,300 milligrams a day. Unfortunately, if you eat out a lot, or use a great deal of processed food products, that number adds up pretty quickly, even if you never touch a salt shaker. Keep in mind that the more highly-processed a food is, the more sodium you'll usually see. So it's a good idea to limit those processed foods as much as possible and gravitate to low-sodium or no-sodium items when given a choice.

So you see how confusing all of this can be. Don't you wish there was an easier way to determine whether or not a food is or isn't a good choice? Well, there is.

Download the app Fooducate at <u>www.fooducate.com</u>. You can take pictures of the bar codes on your favorite foods, and you'll get a rating—anywhere from A+ to D-. And there's even a feature to look for alternatives with higher grades.

The exciting news is that this may be the future for labeling foods. Currently, there is legislation in process advocating for the use of this grading system by food manufacturers to make it easier for consumers. But for now, we'll need to use our smartphones to do so. Yes, it takes time, but once you have a list of the products that are the best for you, food shopping will be a breeze. And remember, incremental changes lead to great results.

FOOD FOR THOUGHT...
QUESTIONS & REFLECTIONS

1. How often do you read food labels before choosing a brand at the market?

    Never   _____

    Rarely   _____

    Occasionally   _____

    Often   _____

    Always   _____

2. How clearly do you understand what you see on food labels?

    Not at all   _____

    A little   _____

    For the most part   _____

    Very well   _____

3. What are you willing to do the next time you grocery shop that will help you use food labels to make wiser choices around some of the packaged foods you regularly buy?

ACTION STEPS & EXERCISES

1. Educate yourself on reading food labels and practice doing so when shopping.

2. When reading food labels, pay close attention to serving sizes.

3. Take note of additives and words on labels that are multisyllabic, and that you can't pronounce. Note words ending in "-ose." Choose products that have fewer ingredients in general, less additives and unpronounceable ingredients, and that are low in sugar and high in fiber.

4. Ask your doctor if there are any ingredients you should limit or avoid.

5. Download the Fooducate app on your smartphone and try using it the next time you grocery shop. Choose a time to do so when you aren't overly rushed.

TIP #18

Avoid buying trigger foods that you know will cause you to lose control and overeat. Keep them out of your home and office.

This week's tip seems so obvious to me. If you know you have difficulty controlling yourself around certain foods, why would you buy them? Although I've heard it a million times, it still astounds me when a client says,

"But I should be able to control myself. It's not fair for me to keep those foods out of my house and deprive my family just because I can't stop eating them."

Would you leave the dog biscuits on the coffee table where they can be gobbled up by your dog because you've "trained" him not to steal food? Or would you tell a recovered alcoholic to leave the vodka sitting on the counter where it can be seen each day because he/she *should* be able to control him- or herself? Come on... Let's get real.

When we're trying to avoid temptation of any kind, it's a lot easier when it is not around. That's why they say, "Out of sight, out of mind." The inability to control yourself in the face of highly tempting treats is not a personality flaw. It's human! And why would you make this weight loss journey more difficult than it already is? When you want to travel to a destination, do you take the super highway or the bumpy, unpaved roads?

Losing weight is hard. Food temptation is everywhere—the supermarket checkout line, the gas station, and even the local hardware store where there's candy for sale at the front counter. So why, oh why, would you make it available in your home where you have a choice in the matter?

As for the family members of your household, you're not being a wonderful spouse, parent, or roommate by continuously buying those goodies because you know they enjoy them. There are a lot of other ways to show you care. Each time you purchase those foods while telling yourself you will resist, you set yourself up for failure. Really consider your actions. Who are you kidding?

For example, if ice cream is your weakness, it shouldn't

be in your home. Having quarts of that treat in the freezer will result in the ice cream calling your name every time you walk by the fridge. If your family wants ice cream, take them to the local store where they can purchase some. If you decide to treat yourself, your purchase will be portion controlled. As long as you've figured it into your daily calorie count, go for it.

I'm going to share my weakness with you. It's pretzels! Actually, anything salty and crunchy can easily cause me to lose control. Pretzels, pita chips, or even crackers. I just can't seem to stop once I start eating them. So I just don't buy these snacks. If I do purchase any, it means I have company coming to visit. Then the bag gets opened when they arrive, and any leftovers get dumped when the company leaves.

Now, that's not to say I don't occasionally enjoy pretzels. I do love them, especially those honey mustard flavored ones! But, if I find myself craving them, I *plan* to have some. I buy the very best brand in a small, portion-controlled size, and totally enjoy when I indulge. And that's what I recommend you do as well.

Stop placing those "out-of-control food temptations" in your home. When you truly crave and desire them, you'll have to work a little hard to get them. You'll need to leave the comfort of your home to go and purchase a small, portion-controlled amount of the best quality you can buy. Savor the flavor, take pleasure in the taste, and then be done with it.

So I ask you, "What's the one food that shows up in your home way too often that you really can't stop eating once you start?" **Commit to stop buying it. Make it off limits in your abode.**

You just might be shocked at the number of calories

that easily disappear from your daily input. And that will lead to weight loss. Remember that small changes lead to huge results!

FOOD FOR THOUGHT...
QUESTIONS & REFLECTIONS

1. List your trigger foods, those that you struggle to stop eating once you've started.

   _____

   _____

   _____

   _____

2. Which trigger foods are you committed to no longer purchase or bring into your home?

   _____

   _____

   _____

   _____

ACTION STEPS & EXERCISES

1. Create your shopping list with a conscious plan to omit trigger foods.

2. Commit to getting rid of all trigger foods in your home. Throw or give them away. Just clear your kitchen of the temptations you cannot resist.

3. If you can't bear the thought of getting rid of food you already have, look at the portion sizes. Dole out enough for one serving for yourself at one sitting. For example, separate pretzels or cookies by placing them on a plate, napkin, or in a baggie, and hide the rest of the package away, out of sight.

4. Talk to your family members about what foods you'll no longer buy regularly, and explain why. Assure them that, if they want a particular treat, you can take them out (or they can go themselves) to pick up portion-controlled snacks of that sort.

TIP #19

Drink water before meals.

I'm very excited to share this tip with you: **Drink an eight-ounce glass of water or two before every meal.** You might already know that drinking more water can be a helpful tool when weight loss is a goal and have probably heard plenty of explanations as to why. If you use water to replace sugar-laden drinks, like soda, sweetened teas, juices, or lemonade, you're going to be cutting back on a significant amount of calories. However, if you've already eliminated those unnecessary calories from your daily input, and you're not drinking excess calories, does increasing your water intake make a difference?

Water has been touted to boost your metabolism, suppress your appetite and, ironically, to flush out excess water weight. If you're bloated, drinking water will decrease the bloating. This idea sounds counterintuitive, but for most people it's true.

Now, what about this idea of drinking a glass of water before a meal? The intention is that your stomach will feel fuller; you'll be a little less hungry and will potentially eat fewer calories. I know many clients who find this strategy to be helpful. So do I. Until quite recently, there was little research to back up these claims.

Will drinking water before meals actually lead to additional weight loss? Well, here is some exciting research that emerged this very year from the University of Birmingham in the UK. The results were published recently in the Journal of Obesity. Researchers took 84 obese individuals and divided them into two groups. Both groups received a weight management consultation that covered lifestyle changes, healthier diet choices, the benefits of more exercise, plus additional information that health care professionals often suggest to people to help them along their weight loss journeys. One group was specifically instructed to drink 16 ounces of water before meals, and the other was told to imagine feeling full approximately 30 minutes before eating a meal.

Twelve weeks later, the water drinkers—those who drank water 30 minutes before the meal—lost an average of 2.87 pounds. That's almost three pounds more than those who just imagined that they were full. Individuals who just drank water before a meal once a day, or not at all, lost an average of 1.76 pounds. But those folks who drank 16 ounces of water before all three meals each day lost an average of 9.48 pounds, clearly more than the first group. Wow, 9.5 lbs! How impressive is that? Here we have scientific evidence that drinking water does fill up your tummy and makes you feel fuller and less hungry.

What do you think? Is this a strategy you'd like to try? If so, keep in mind that, if you do drink water before a meal in the hopes of enhancing weight loss, you still need to pay attention to what and how much you're eating. Drinking water before a meal with an unhealthy plate full of calorie-rich foods won't give you the results you're hoping for. So, drink a full glass of water or two before each meal. Make sure the meal is comprised of healthy, clean, and nourishing foods, and eat enough to satisfy yourself without feeling stuffed. You just may find that this is a super easy and cost-effective tool in your weight loss toolbox.

Do you want to experiment this week? I hope so, because I am passionate about spreading the message I often repeat: If you want to lose weight, don't go on a diet, because small lifestyle shifts bring about significant changes that will benefit you physically and psychologically.

FOOD FOR THOUGHT...
QUESTIONS & REFLECTIONS

1. On average, how much water do you think you drink each day? When do you typically reach for a glass?

   _____

   _____

2. Which, if any, high-calorie/sugar-laden beverages do you often consume with meals or other times of the day?

   _____

   _____

   _____

3. On a scale of 1–10, with 1=not at all, and 10=totally, how committed are you to replacing the beverages you listed above with water? How do you feel about the number you chose?

   _____

   _____

   _____

4. What can you do to support your efforts to drink a glass of water before each meal? How will you remember to do so?

_____

_____

_____

_____

_____

_____

_____

ACTION STEPS & EXERCISES

1. If you drink sugar- and calorie-rich beverages, check the labels for the total number of calories per serving for each. Write it down next to the drinks you listed above.

2. Begin to rid your home of them completely, decide to no longer purchase them, and gradually wean yourself off those unnecessary calories.

3. Choose one meal to focus on this week. Commit to drinking eight ounces of water before that meal each day. When that behavior feels like a habit, choose to focus on the second meal. Continue to do so until you have established a routine of

drinking at least one glass of water before every meal.

4. Implement a once- or twice-a-week weigh-in plan (which we'll discuss in Tip #21). Chart your weight while you experiment with drinking water before meals and eliminate high-calorie/sugar-laden beverages from your day.

5. Bonus: Keep track of the money you save when you eat out and no longer order drinks like soda, sweetened teas, juices, or lemonade.

TIP #20

Drink lots of clear liquids all day—primarily water, seltzer, or tea.

Do you know the signs of dehydration? You probably think they include feeling exceptionally thirsty, lightheaded or dizzy, with a headache, nausea, or the shakes. And you'd be right. Those are some of the signs of extreme dehydration, but you could be dehydrated and not experience any of those symptoms.

Mild dehydration often goes unnoticed in most adults. As a matter of fact, once you feel thirsty, you're probably already mildly dehydrated.

So what does this have to do with weight loss? Well, did you know that dehydration often masks itself as hunger? Sometimes you notice a sensation that you mistake for hunger when your body just needs some liquids. If you respond inappropriately, or in other words, by eating rather than drinking, you'll be taking in excess calories. Unless the foods you choose are high in water content, such as watermelon, grapefruit, cucumbers, lettuce, or clear broths, those extra calories won't rehydrate you and may not be necessary if it's not the time for a meal or snack.

Tip #19 explained why water is so good for you and how drinking a full glass of water before each meal has been proven to expedite weight loss. If you are also adding clear liquids to your diet in between meals, you'll reap all the health benefits, avoid dehydration, and help keep your tummy feeling full. And that can result in a decrease of overall caloric intake at the end of the day, which is the key to weight loss. Despite all the tricks, tools, exercises, and other factors you incorporate during a weight loss journey, if you are not in a caloric deficit (that is, taking in fewer calories than your body burns), the number on the scale will not go down.

So you might be wondering how to implement the simple idea of taking in more liquids. You will need to develop a new habit of drinking lots of water, tea, seltzer, and other clear liquids throughout the day. As with all habits, adding a cue is helpful. What that means is that you create reminders for yourself: "When I do this, then I do that." Let me give you some examples: When I wake in the morning, I drink the glass of water I left by my bedside. When starting dinner preparation, I put a large glass of seltzer on the counter as I am taking the dinner ingredients out of the fridge. When I begin work in the morning, I bring a full water bottle and place it on my office desk. When I check emails, I sip from my water bottle. When I make my lunch, I take a glass of unsweetened ice tea (or hot herbal tea depending on the season) to enjoy with my midday meal.

I'm sure you get the gist. Now it's a matter of applying the awareness and strategies that will increase your liquid intake and subsequently decrease your weight.

FOOD FOR THOUGHT... QUESTIONS & REFLECTIONS

1. What clear liquids to you usually keep handy at home, work, etc.?

   _____

   _____

   _____

2. What cues might you set up that could help you form the habit of drinking clear liquids throughout the day? (Try to create when/then rules to follow. For example: When I wake in the morning, then I drink a full glass of water.)

   _____

   _____

   _____

   _____

   _____

   _____

   _____

ACTION STEPS & EXERCISES

1. This week, when you notice signs of fatigue, foggy brain, headache or slight light-headedness, drink some clear liquid (water, seltzer, tea, or broth) before reaching for food. Reevaluate how you feel after a few minutes.

2. Choose one of your "when/then" rules from above, and commit to practicing it this week.

3. Slowly work on developing new habits of drinking more clear liquids, perhaps beginning with water, at set times during the day. Don't wait until you notice that you are thirsty before reaching for liquids.

4. Make sure to have these hydrating liquids available no matter where you live, work, or play.

TIP #21

Weigh in at least once a week. Ignorance is not bliss when it comes to weight loss.

In the very many years I have been working with weight loss clients, two dominant behaviors stand out when it comes to stepping on the scale. One is complete avoidance, and the other is obsession—weighing in every day or even several times a day.

In my opinion, neither one is helpful. Let's talk about avoidance first.

So often, individuals decide they need to lose weight, not because they step on the scale and see a number that takes them by surprise, but rather because some other impetus for change occurs. You might notice how uncomfortable your clothing fits; everyday activities leave you tired or breathless; maybe your knees start hurting; perhaps a doctor or spouse comments on your weight; or you look at a picture of yourself and say, "Oh my gosh, I hadn't realized how heavy I've gotten!"

Whatever the driving force, it becomes your motivation to make some behavioral shifts. Perhaps you start exercising or watching your food choices, like swearing off bread and wine. The thought behind this is, "When I feel lighter, I'll step on the scale. Let me just take some weight off first." You simply don't want to know what the scale reads—it's too daunting. The problem is that when it comes to weight loss, ignorance is NOT bliss! It can be a hindrance to success.

How will you know if the efforts you are making are paying off if you do not have a starting point and check-in points? You may think you only need to lose five pounds to achieve a healthy body weight, but it might actually be 15. That information just may alter your approach and efforts.

Another common occurrence I see happens even after you have successfully taken off some weight. Avoiding the scale when you go off track until you feel like you are back on track is a recipe for disaster! The reality check of knowing how far off you've gone from your "happy weight range" can be the motivation to get you back on track sooner rather than later.

Let's look at the opposite extreme, obsessive weighing.

Rather than never stepping on the scale, some folks are incessantly jumping on it. There are so many problems with this approach; I barely know where to begin. For too many people, and possibly you as well, the scale is an emotional trigger—the number you see can make or break your day. When it is good news, you feel great about yourself, you are happy, you have a sense of well-being, and it motivates you to stay on track. When it is bad news, you plummet into a downward spiral. You start saying things to yourself that you would never say to your best friend, such as, "I'm a complete failure. I have no will power. This isn't worth all of the hard work. I'm destined to be fat." And on and on and on. The mood you are left in can influence your choices for the rest of the day. Negativity leads to poor decision making and low motivation.

The second problem with continuously jumping on the scale is that your body weight constantly fluctuates from day to day or even within the same day. Weight variations are normal, and they happen to everybody. They can be caused by many different factors, such as consumption of a big meal, excess salt intake, water retention, constipation, and hormonal changes. But even if you know this logically, fluctuations on the scale can be very frustrating, and they can cause you to lose hope when it comes to losing weight.

One more reason I dislike the daily weigh-in approach is that it keeps you focused on the number as the reward instead of the changes regarding how you look and feel. Weight reduction should be about much more than reaching a particular number on the scale. The process should center upon eating well, becoming healthy and active, and feeling better both physically and emotionally overall.

Let's take a reality check when it comes to weighing in. The number on the scale is not a judge as to whether you are a good person or a bad person. It has absolutely nothing to do with your character, strengths, or weaknesses. It is just information! When it comes to your weight loss journey, the scale should be your GPS. It tells you if you are on the right road toward your destination or if you need to recalculate. And that's it!

What is the best schedule for weighing in? I have found that what works for my clients is stepping on the scale either once or twice a week and charting the information. Begin by graphing your starting weight and continue to chart each time you weigh in so that over time you can see a direction of change. That way, when you notice an increase (which absolutely will happen, as I pointed out above), although disappointing, you will eventually discern a pattern. That will be a downward trend for those who are making positive changes in their nutritional habits and physical activity levels. For individuals who choose to weigh themselves twice a week and there is a weight increase, they feel better knowing they will not wait an entire week before checking in again. **Regardless of whether it's once or twice a week, I do recommend weighing in on the same day, time of day, mode of dress, and using the same scale.**

FOOD FOR THOUGHT...
QUESTIONS & REFLECTIONS

1. Do you fit into the "avoidance" or "obsessive" habit of weighing in? In either case, what is the reasoning behind your approach?

   _____

   _____

   _____

   _____

2. Describe how you respond emotionally to fluctuations in your weight when you step on the scale. How might charting your weight once or twice a week help you to accomplish your goals?

   _____

   _____

   _____

   _____

ACTION STEPS & EXERCISES

1. If you do not already own one, purchase a high-quality scale this week. See the recommendations in Appendix C.

2. Think about what suits you most. Do you want to weigh in once a week, or twice? Pick one or two days of the week when you will routinely weigh in.

3. Print out a copy of the weight chart in Appendix B and begin tracking your weekly weigh-ins.

4. Aside from seeing a change in the number on your scale, what are the benefits you hope to realize by losing weight? List them below. See if you can come up with at least ten!

TIP #22

Have a happy target weight to strive for, with a five-pound acceptable weight range.

Most people have a specific number in mind when they embark on a weight loss journey. What's your goal weight? Perhaps it is what you weighed in college, on your wedding day, your pre-baby weight, or the number you remember weighing when you felt thrilled with your body. Sadly, this is often an unrealistic number.

Striving for it can be discouraging and disappointing. It can keep you from appreciating the positive changes you do accomplish, because those just don't feel good enough.

So how should you decide what *is* the target weight to strive for? The answer to that question is going to be unique to you. Let me give you some guidelines to help you determine what goal is realistic. *No matter what that number turns out to be,* I encourage you to establish a weight *range* instead of a very specific number that spells success.

In Tip #21, we noted how fickle the scale is and how day-to-day changes are normal and to be expected. So having a very concrete number in mind can leave you celebrating one day and discouraged the next. When you have a five-pound range—that is, two up and two down from your happy target number—your weight loss goal is to reach that range *and* sustain it over time.

First, let me help you decide on a realistic, happy weight rather than choosing a number from long ago that just might not be possible anymore. You can establish your *range* based on that figure. (No pun intended.)

The following describes several methods that you can use to land on a goal weight that is realistic uniquely to you:

Can you recall a *recent* time (within the past few years) when you weighed less than your current weight, and you sustained it for an extended period, at least six months to a year? A weight you were able to *maintain* without a highly restrictive diet plan and punishing exercise routine? A time when you were feeling a lot more comfortable in your body than you are now? That should become your happy weight.

You'll want to take a different approach to determining a target weight if you are very overweight, and either sense or have been told by a health care provider that the extra pounds are putting your health at risk. Your doctor may or may not have advised a specific body weight for you to get to, and it is always a good idea to ask for guidance. However, the two methods I am about to show you are often how health care providers arrive at that number.

Your body mass index (BMI) is based on your height and weight. It's a useful tool to help measure body fat and gauge your chances of disease. Many health care professionals suggest that you learn your BMI and, if it is high, you make efforts to lose enough weight so that you fall into the healthy range. However, the BMI isn't a foolproof number. If you're muscular, the BMI can overstate your body fat. If you're older and have less muscle mass, it can understate your body fat. If you're interested in determining your BMI, refer to the resources available in Appendix B.

In my opinion, your waist size can give you a better picture of your health—especially if you're muscular. To measure your waistline, simply take a tape measure and put it around your middle, just above your hip bones. (For a detailed description of how to measure waist circumference, go to Appendix B.) A waist size over 35 inches for a woman and 40 inches for a man means it's time to take action. This is especially the case if that number is coupled with other health risk factors, such as high blood pressure, high cholesterol, triglycerides, or blood glucose levels, and/or an extremely sedentary lifestyle.

A steady stream of research has found that as little as a 10-percent reduction in total body weight can make a significant positive impact on your health profile. So that's a great objective to work toward.

Then what is the target number if you choose to lose 10 percent of your current weight? Let's say that, at present, you weigh 180 pounds. A 10-percent loss would equal 18 pounds, bringing you to 162 pounds. Now, let's create a range: Add two pounds and subtract two pounds, and your range becomes 160–164 pounds. Once you fall into that range and sustain it comfortably over time, you can decide if it is necessary and you are motivated to strive for another 10-percent decrease.

One last point about maintenance. Once you've reached that happy weight range, consider the higher number of the two (164 pounds in the example we used) entirely acceptable. If the scale tips above it, swing into action immediately. Check in on the habits you were practicing while losing weight or remaining within the range, and you'll probably figure out where you've slipped. Get back on track, and very soon you'll be within that happy range once more.

Now you have another strategy to advance you on the path to weight loss and maintenance. Adjust your mindset and ascertain your five-pound acceptable weight range. Quickly leap into action when the scale exceeds the highest number in that range.

You'll likely feel relieved to consider a *range* rather than aiming for one specific number on the scale. Perhaps this will inspire you even more to begin or further your weight loss journey.

FOOD FOR THOUGHT...
QUESTIONS & REFLECTIONS

1. Do you have a particular body weight that you have been hoping to reach? After reading this tip, would you say it is realistic?

   Yes _____ No _____

2. Was there ever a time in your life when you felt satisfied and happy with your weight?

   Yes _____ No _____

   If yes, how much did you weigh at that time?

   _____

   When was that?

   _____

   How long were you able to maintain that weight?

   _____

3. Reflect on your current weight and where you'd like to be in the future. What is the one action you are willing to take right now that will support you reaching your happy target range in the future?

   _____

ACTION STEPS & EXERCISES

1. Review the several methods described above and decide which you will implement to determine your happy target weight and range. Create your realistic five-pound target weight range and write it down.

2. When you look at the range you created above, how does it make you feel?

_____

_____

_____

_____

_____

3. On a scale of 1–10, how confident are you that you can reach that range and maintain it? (1=not at all, 10=totally confident.) If you're at 6 or less, what would you need to do to increase your confidence level?

_____

_____

_____

_____

_____

_____

_____

TIP #23

Strength train at least twice a week for a minimum of 20 minutes.

There are numerous reasons as to why it is a good idea to incorporate strength training into your weekly exercise schedule. Strength training builds strong and toned muscles, which makes everything you do in your daily life—such as climbing stairs, carrying groceries, lifting your children or grandchildren, and so much more—easier. And let's be honest; a muscular and toned body looks better in clothing and in the mirror.

However, strength training yields benefits that go well beyond the appearance of nicely toned muscles. Those include enhanced balance, coordination, flexibility, and posture. Improvements in balance and flexibility can reduce your risk of falling by as much as 40 percent. And that is certainly crucial as we age!

After puberty, whether you are a man or a woman, you begin to lose approximately one percent of bone and muscle strength every year. To stop, reverse, and even prevent those deficits, you will want to add strength training to your workouts. Weightlifting stresses your bones (in a good way), which in turn increases bone density and reduces the risk of osteoporosis.

If you have arthritis, strength training can be as effective as medication in diminishing arthritis pain. It has been proven to help post-menopausal women increase bone density and lower the risk of bone fractures. And for the 14 million Americans with type 2 diabetes, strength training, along with other healthy lifestyle adjustments, can help improve glucose control.

It has also been established that lifting weights elevates your endorphin level, which will boost your mood and confidence. Strength training has even been shown to be a great antidepressant, to help you sleep better, and to improve your overall quality of life.

Strength training is not just for body builders; it can benefit just about everyone. And it is particularly important for those who are trying to lose weight.

Every cell in our bodies, including muscle and fat cells, require energy (fuel from food) to do its job and function properly. When we take in an excess, it gets stored as fat. Since muscle is more metabolically active than fat, it requires more calories just to exist. The more muscle you have, the more calories you will burn, even when you are asleep! The reason for this is that more calories are used to form and maintain muscle than are used to add fat. In fact, strength training can boost your metabolism by 15 percent, and that can *really* jump-start a weight loss plan. You not only burn calories while you're lifting weights, but your body also continues to burn even more calories after your session ends.

So strength training aids in *shedding pounds*, and it also helps *maintain weight loss*. A recent study revealed that women who followed a weight training routine three times a week increased the number of calories burned during regular daily activity, which helped them maintain their current weight over time.

If I have convinced you that strength training should be part of your weight loss *and* healthy lifestyle toolbox, how should you begin? If you are new to weightlifting or have not exercised in this manner for a long time, it might be a good idea to enlist the help of a fitness professional. Most gyms offer a no-cost orientation to the weight room and even a complimentary session with a trainer. Hiring a professional for one or two additional strength training sessions can help you develop a program you can then follow on your own.

If you would rather lift at home, you can purchase hand weights and an exercise mat at minimal cost. There are many excellent instructional DVDs and online content available to help you learn proper form and technique. And the instructors on these videos tend to be highly motivating. I love the video series offered by the Mayo Clinic, which you can find on their website: www.mayoclinic.org/healthy-lifestyle/fitness/in-depth/strength-training/art-20046031.

Of course, as with any new exercise endeavor, **check with your health care provider to ensure that you do not have any medical conditions that would prevent you from strength training.** You can start slowly by adding a few minutes of strength training to your current routine, and continue to build upon it as your confidence in your form and ability grows.

FOOD FOR THOUGHT... QUESTIONS & REFLECTIONS

1. On a scale of 1–10 (1=not at all, 10=totally committed), how committed are you to incorporating strength training into your weekly routine? If your commitment level is a 6 or lower, what would you need to do in order to increase your commitment/motivation to a higher level?

   _____
   _____
   _____
   _____
   _____

2. If you're not already doing so, how best could you learn proper form and technique for strength exercises and develop a routine that is safe for you?

   _____
   _____

_____

_____

_____

3. Having read the above tip, what benefits to strength training are most motivating for you?

_____

_____

_____

4. Which environment is the most intriguing to you for incorporating a strength training routine; at a gym, at a class, in a specialized studio, or home; with free weights, machines, or using your own body weight?

_____

_____

_____

ACTION STEPS & EXERCISES

1. Review your current exercise regimen and daily schedule. Plan how to incorporate strength training into your weekly routine.

2. Experiment with strength training at least twice a week for a minimum of 20 minutes each session.

3. Investigate low-cost or free gym/trainer orientations near to where you live or work. Consider enlisting the help of a personal trainer, at least until you learn the exercises.

4. If you like the idea of strength training at home rather than in a gym or studio, peruse, choose, and use some of the many instructional DVDs or strength training workouts you can find on the internet.

TIP #24

Do 30 minutes of aerobic exercise at least five days each week.

If, at present, you are not working out on a regular basis, you might find this to be one of the most challenging of all the tips so far. In all likelihood, your schedule is already overloaded, so trying to figure out where you can add 30 minutes of aerobic exercise into your daily schedule for five days a week is daunting! However, read along and you will better understand how to accomplish this and why it can be an integral part of weight loss and maintenance, not to mention all of the other wonderful benefits of aerobic exercise.

First, I want to emphasize the good news: *You will not have to do the day's 30 minutes of aerobic exercise all at once.* In fact, the most recent research finds that breaking up your workout into smaller sessions—for example, three 10-minute sessions a day—is just as beneficial as a consistent 30 minutes.

The American College of Sports Medicine guidelines recommend accumulating 150 minutes of moderate-intensity exercise or 75 minutes of vigorous-intensity exercise a week to prevent chronic disease. I am sure I don't need to list the myriad of health benefits that have been scientifically proven to result from regular exercise. (In fact, I covered several of those in Tip #23.) And if losing weight and sustaining a target weight (or weight range) are important goals to you, exercise should be a priority.

When it comes to losing weight, the most critical element that will determine your success is what you eat. But adding exercise to your regimen will jump-start a weight reduction program and is *essential* for maintenance once you reach your goal. The National Weight Control Registry is an ongoing research study that includes people (18 years or older) who have lost at least 30 pounds and kept them off for a minimum of one year. Members complete annual questionnaires regarding their current weight, diet and exercise habits, and behavioral strategies for weight loss maintenance. 90 percent of the participants exercise for an average of one hour per day.

This tip recommends 30 minutes of aerobic exercise a day, but now I'm providing statistics that indicate sustained weight loss requires one hour a day! Have I overwhelmed you? I don't mean to do so, but this information is important for you to know and understand, since sustained weight loss is what you are aspiring to.

Essentially, the overall issue I'm highlighting is that most of us are too sedentary in our normal daily routines. The advantages of the technological age have taken a serious toll on our need for movement, and thus the number of calories we burn during the course of the day has dwindled dramatically. In modern times, then, we need to thoughtfully and proactively incorporate more physical activity into our days.

Most of us claim that we simply do not have a chance to fit in exercise. Surveys indicate that the average American watches three and one-half hours of TV a day. We surf the internet, play games on our cell phones, and visit social media sites daily. We make time for our manicures and hair appointments. We meet friends for coffee, lunch, or dinner. Sure, those activities are important, and I am not suggesting you forgo all of them. However, the real question concerning integrating exercise is not how to do it, but rather how much of a priority it is to us.

If you decide that weight reduction and good health are valuable, you will find the time to exercise! If fitting in a full 30 minutes seems too overwhelming, ask yourself, "Where can I find a few minutes several times a day to take a break and move?" You can walk the dog after breakfast; climb the stairs rather than take the elevator; park on the opposite side of the mall from where you will be shopping; meet your friends at the running (or walking) track rather than at the cafe; or take a dance class on the weekends.

Start slowly and build as time goes on. You just might discover that you begin to look forward to your activity breaks. As you now know—if you did not before—exercise isn't only a great calorie burner, but also a super way to relieve stress and lift your mood. Why not give it a try? Commit yourself to incorporating exercise into each day as part of your new weight loss regimen along the path of improved well-being.

FOOD FOR THOUGHT...
QUESTIONS & REFLECTIONS

1. How would you describe your current lifestyle regarding your activity level?

   _____

   _____

   _____

   _____

   _____

2. What, if any, physical activities and exercise are part of your day-to-day life?

   _____

   _____

   _____

   _____

   _____

3. What are your primary motivators to begin an exercise program, or to remain consistent if you're already exercising?

_____

_____

_____

_____

_____

4. If you currently engage in an aerobic activity at least 30 minutes a day, what benefits have you experienced? If you're not consistently exercising, what benefits would you hope to achieve if you embark on a physical activity program?

_____

_____

_____

5. What aerobic activities can you add to your daily routine to amp up your weight loss efforts?

_____

_____

6. On a scale of 1–10, how committed are you to beginning and/or maintaining a consistent aerobic exercise routine for at least 30 minutes a day, five times a week?

_____

ACTION STEPS & EXERCISES

1. If you haven't been exercising on a regular basis, or plan to significantly increase the level of exercise you currently do, discuss your intentions with your personal physician before embarking on a new program.

2. Experiment with incorporating aerobic activity for at least 30 minutes for several days this week, even if you don't do it all in one session. Write down how you feel on the days you exercise and any changes related to your weight loss journey. For the next several weeks, add on another day until you're working out aerobically at least five days each week.

3. If you don't already have a membership, consider joining a health club close to your home or office. Take advantage of trial memberships and free training in the beginning.

4. If you can't join a gym and haven't done aerobic exercise before, seek out instructional DVDs or online videos, at least to start you on this part of your weight loss journey.

TIP #25

When short on time, squeeze in a quick workout rather than not at all. A little exercise is always better than no exercise.

Is consistent physical activity already a part of your lifestyle? If so, have you ever planned to exercise, for example first thing in the morning or right after work, but then got derailed? It's entirely possible that you have incorporated exercise into your day's schedule, yet for one reason or another, that workout never comes to fruition.

Some mornings, you tell yourself you will go to the gym straight from work. As you walk toward the door, though, your coworker asks for a minute of your time. You stop to be polite, listen, give some advice or help him/her figure out a problem, and finally leave for the day. When you look at the clock, you begin to think, "Now I don't have enough time for a workout." Perhaps you were aiming for the 6:00 p.m. spinning class and now you'll be too late. You usually spend an hour spinning, but that coworker ate up 25 minutes of your time. Then you ask yourself, "Why bother going at all?" Or maybe you intended to take an hour-long walk with the dog before dinner, and now you only have 20 minutes. You figure, "What's the point?" Right?

If I skipped a workout on every occasion this kind of scenario played out, I would probably exercise 50 percent less than the amount of time I currently do. Time is such a precious commodity and it seems to slip away so quickly. Although we often rely on schedules, our activities frequently last longer than we planned, the unexpected happens, or we become so wrapped up in our current tasks that we do not take note of the time.

Here is the opportunity to alter your thought process, particularly the "I-don't-have-enough-time-so-why-bother?" refrain. Because the truth is that *a short workout is always better than no workout*.

In an ideal world, we would preplan our exercise sessions and set alarms to remind ourselves to stop what we are doing and go work out. But we don't live in a perfect world. We live in the real world and, therefore, we need to adjust our expectations as such.

We need to shift our mindsets toward the notion that whatever movement and exercise we can fit in is better than not exercising at all. Short bursts of activity do add up in terms of their physical and emotional health benefits.

There are many options when it comes to incorporating exercise despite the demands of a busy week, holiday seasons, or common sidetracks.

You can break down each exercise session into several shorter periods; for example, three 10-minute bouts rather than a full 30 minutes, as emphasized in Tip #24. Or when time-crunched, as long as you have no medical restrictions, you can increase the intensity of a curtailed workout. A higher-intensity session for 20 minutes will reap the same, if not more, benefits than the moderate-intensity 30-minute sessions. A brisk 20-minute walk will burn more calories than not walking at all, even if you had planned a 45-minute workout.

What should be gleaned from Tip #25 is that every time you choose working out or any movement over a stationary activity, you burn more calories, keep your metabolism revved, and reinforce the habit of exercising. And that is the ultimate goal: **to cultivate or perpetuate the habit of exercising most days of the week, even when you can't complete a full session.** So begin moving and ditch the excuses. The next time you hear that inner voice say, "Why bother?" remind yourself that consistent workouts—extensive or brief—accumulate to promote weight loss and multiple health benefits as well. Enjoy your regular workouts, no matter how long they last. Look toward the future when they become part of your regular routine and less of a challenge.

FOOD FOR THOUGHT... QUESTIONS & REFLECTIONS

1. What are the primary reasons you don't exercise consistently or miss preplanned workouts?

   _____

   _____

   _____

   _____

   _____

   _____

   _____

   _____

2. How often do you find yourself "skipping" a planned exercise session because you have run out of time?

   _____

   _____

3. What deterrents or distractions get in the way, causing you to skip a scheduled workout?

_____

_____

_____

_____

_____

_____

_____

4. Thus far, what have you believed the duration an exercise session "should" be that would make it worthwhile? What might you tell yourself to change that perception the next time you decide you don't have enough time for a prearranged workout?

_____

_____

_____

_____

ACTION STEPS & EXERCISES

1. Make the conscious decision to exercise daily, regardless of the length of the session.

2. Review each day's schedule and think about where you can fit in a workout, even if it's only for a few minutes at a time.

3. In those instances when you are sidetracked and run late, commit to exercising for as long as you have left during your pre-designated time frame.

TIP #26

Schedule exercise into your calendar in advance and treat it like a business appointment. Non-negotiable!

Before we dive into Tip #26, I want to congratulate you! If you've been following my tips chronologically, adding them to your toolbox one week at a time, you've made it to the halfway mark. You have read and hopefully implemented 25 tips to help you lose weight *or* maintain your healthy weight, all without going on a diet.

Before reviewing this newest tip, briefly pause to reflect upon what has changed for you in the past few months. What new habits have you established that are helping you reach your weight reduction goal—habits that you had not formed over recent years? What challenges are you still facing?

Take a few moments to journal your answers to the above questions. Acknowledge the successes you've had so far. It's easy to forget accomplishments when the destination may still seem far off. I don't want that to happen for you. Every new habit that helps solidify a healthier lifestyle is worth celebrating!

Now we can take a closer look at this chapter, Tip #26: **Schedule exercise by adding it to your calendar in advance. Treat it as if it was a business appointment and make it non-negotiable.**

Have you ever heard the expression "what gets calendared gets done"? How often do you think about something you want to do, loosely plan when you'll do it (without writing it down), and then somehow never get around to it? This certainly happens to me. If I don't schedule important activities on my calendar, I either forget about them completely or something "urgent" redirects my attention.

Well, exercise is no different. If you value exercise and recognize its worth, then you must schedule it into your days. If you're already at a point where you consider yourself a regular, lifetime exerciser—in other words, you consistently work out three, four, or even five times a week— you probably don't need to schedule your sessions onto your calendar. I would bet, though, that any routine exerciser knows in advance when he/she will be working out each day.

However, if you're inconsistent with your workouts, exercise will never become a habit unless you begin pre-scheduling and adding it to your calendar. *And* you must treat exercise "appointments" with the same level of priority that you would a business meeting.

I've already shared with you that when it comes to weight loss, although exercise helps, hands down, what you eat is the ultimate key to success. Nevertheless, when you reach your goal weight and turn your attention toward maintenance, exercise is essential. So the sooner you get into the habit of regularly working out, the better your chances will become of sustaining that weight loss and keeping within your target weight range. As much as I wish it weren't so, it becomes more difficult to sustain a stable weight as we age. Regular exercisers will have a much easier time preventing pounds from creeping up as the years go by.

Also, I have heard hundreds of clients and friends tell me that when they are exercising regularly, they are much more in control of their food intake. It seems easier to stay on track with a healthy eating plan when daily workouts are consistent.

Let's get back to the idea of treating exercise as one would a business appointment. I'm pretty sure that you wouldn't cancel a business commitment unless an actual emergency arose. Even if you were tired; even if your favorite show was on TV; or even if your best friend called.

Perhaps you're thinking, "I have too much work to do to take the time to exercise." Allow me to share the results of a study completed at Stockholm University and it just might change your mind. Their researchers found that total productivity increased more when employees exercised two and one-half hours per week than when they worked an extra two and one-half hours each week.

So right now, open your calendar. Look at the current week. When can you schedule your next workout? Lock in that time immediately. Make it non-negotiable. If you schedule at least three "appointments" with yourself to exercise at the beginning of each week, in another six months, if not sooner, you will have become a consistent, lifetime exerciser. You will lose—and continue to lose—excess weight more easily than you ever imagined.

FOOD FOR THOUGHT... QUESTIONS & REFLECTIONS

1. If you're not already exercising on a regular basis, what excuses do you tell yourself as to why not? (E.g., not enough time, I hate exercise, it's not necessary for weight loss, etc.)

   _____

   _____

   _____

   _____

   _____

   _____

   _____

2. What would you need to tell yourself in order for consistent exercise to become a priority for you?

   _____

   _____

   _____

_____

_____

_____

_____

3. Do you typically, or have you ever, scheduled exercise into your calendar in advance? What impact does/might doing so have for you?

_____

_____

_____

_____

_____

ACTION STEPS & EXERCISES

1. If you don't already have an appointment calendar, purchase a planner or use an online calendar or phone app into which you will schedule your exercise "appointments." Take a look at the suggested planners in Appendix C.

2. Choose a specific time and day of the week when you will look at your calendar and schedule your exercise appointments.

3. At your designated time each week, plan your exercise appointments and calendar them in.

4. Create reminders for yourself, be they notes or cell phone alerts, before each exercise appointment.

5. If an unexpected and important conflict occurs, immediately reschedule your exercise appointment. Don't let it fall through the cracks and allow yourself to skip it.

6. Check off each scheduled exercise session once you completed it. Doing so will allow you to track your consistency over time and make adjustments, if need be.

TIP #27

Join a group exercise class that is fun and that you will look forward to. If it's gratifying, there's a good chance you will go.

By now you should have a clear understanding of the role exercise plays in losing weight and maintaining your goal weight—or at least keeping within your target range. Nevertheless, if you've never enjoyed exercise, or just don't have much experience working out, you might struggle with the how, when, and where of getting started. A group class could be your answer!

If you choose an activity that feels fun, your chances of sticking with it will increase tremendously. The success of group exercise classes—and the widening range of activities to choose from—happened for a good reason; working out is more enjoyable when you're motivated by a first-rate teacher, exercising with others, and listening to upbeat music. When activities are gratifying, you'll participate in them more often. That certainly makes sense.

Many research studies have indicated that the single most important factor in long-term health and fitness success is one's support system. And where better to find support than in a class filled with like-minded individuals and led by a devoted and knowledgeable instructor? Your classmates plus a caring, dedicated teacher will notice when you don't show up; encourage you when you're feeling unmotivated; joke with you while you both sweat; and basically make the entire workout a lot more fun. Not to mention that, if you have paid in advance (which most gyms and studios require), there's a pretty good chance you will attend. This is likely the case even on days you would rather stay in bed or drive straight home after work rather than going to the gym.

Add that you can choose from so many types of exercise classes. Offerings range from traditional dance-style classes like Jazzercise, Pilates, and Barre, to spinning, kickboxing, or yoga. The list goes on and on. If you bore easily, or the camaraderie of exercising regularly with the same group of people isn't that important to you, look into Class Pass (classpass.com)—a concept that is growing in leaps and bounds in major cities throughout the country. A monthly membership allows you to take as many classes per month as you would like at participating studios, but only visiting the same location up to three times within each month. You can potentially attend a different class every day of the week.

Even though there are fees for taking classes, they don't have to break the budget. Community centers, your local high school, YMCA's, and JCC's usually offer more affordable options than private clubs. With a little extra legwork (no pun intended), you may find discounts, coupons, or even free monthly trials at local gyms and studios.

Nonetheless, if you don't find exercises classes appealing, but there is a particular sport that interests you, perhaps you can sign up for group lessons or club sports. Tennis, golf, soccer, or softball—it doesn't really matter the type of sport. As long as it's an activity that you like and it includes movement, the benefits of the exercise will pay off.

Even equipped with these many suggestions and alternatives, if you still do not find exercise fun, *do it anyway*. **Focus on the benefits of working out:** feeling better and more comfortable in your body, the mood-lifting effect many individuals notice when they finish a satisfying workout, and the fact that you can indulge in buying new clothes for your toned and fit body. Now *that* can be fun!

FOOD FOR THOUGHT... QUESTIONS & REFLECTIONS

1. Do you currently, or have you in the past, participated in exercise classes? What are your overall feelings regarding group fitness classes?

   _____
   _____
   _____
   _____
   _____

2. What options are available for partaking in classes near your work or home?

   _____
   _____
   _____
   _____
   _____
   _____
   _____

3. If you are on a tight budget or prefer not to invest much for exercises classes, what facilities nearby offer low-cost classes, discounts, or trial memberships?

_____

_____

_____

_____

_____

4. If you don't find exercise classes appealing, what sports did you enjoy in the past which you might be open to trying again with group lessons?

_____

_____

_____

_____

_____

ACTION STEPS & EXERCISES

1. Begin researching facilities near to your home and/or workplace that provide exercise classes with the activities you might consider enjoyable. "Research" can include online searches or even asking for word-of-mouth recommendations from friends and family. You can also leverage social media to inquire, e.g. post an ISO (in search of) exercise classes close by.

2. Check out Groupon (groupon.com) and other discount purchasing sites to see if studios in your area offer options for classes that pique your interest. It's a great way to try something new without making a long-term commitment or too much of a financial investment.

3. If you're not keen on exercise in general, reflect on a sport—or sports—you like. Then look into group lessons.

4. Commit to at least trying one or two group classes or lessons. Choose a class and schedule your first session.

TIP #28

*Exercise with a buddy—
a friend or family member.
Commitment to exercise increases
when you partner up.*

Numerous studies demonstrate that social support is strongly associated with exercise adherence. And what could be better than support from an exercise buddy? I often encourage my clients to team up with a friend or family member for workouts and have seen for myself how the "buddy system" helps people maintain exercise consistency.

Since you know exercise plays such an important role in weight loss and maintenance, as well as in your overall health and well-being, it just makes good sense to employ tactics that will aid you in sustaining a regular exercise routine. Working out with others, then, is one more strategy you can use to increase your consistency and, therefore, your success. Those "others" can be the people in a group exercise class, which we already discussed, OR a training partner; your "buddy."

Scheduling an exercise session with another person who depends on you to show up at a pre-determined place and time is an excellent way to ensure you adhere to the plan. If you arranged to work out with an exercise buddy, you're more likely to keep that appointment rather than miss it and let down that friend or family member. Enlisting a training partner keeps you honest and accountable. It eliminates many of the excuses you might make up to skip a session.

An exercise buddy can also encourage you on the days you feel unmotivated. We all have those kinds of days. When you work out side-by-side with another person, you'll push yourself harder than when you work out alone. As a result, your fitness capacity and calorie burning rate increase. That creates a win-win situation for both of you.

Keep in mind that choosing the right buddy is key. You want to make sure this is an individual you will look forward to seeing, enjoy spending time with, and with whom your fitness level is somewhat compatible. If your goal is to one day run a 5K race, but your partner is only interested in a long, slow stroll, you'll be frustrated and unable to fulfill your potential to push yourself further. By the same token, it's also great to exercise with someone whose abilities are slightly superior to yours—a person who will challenge you. However, if they are so much more advanced that you find yourself struggling to keep up, or too exhausted and sore after a partner workout, you might want to rethink that particular exercise alliance.

If you don't know anyone who can partner with you, here are a few ideas: Research local groups of walkers, hikers, runners, or cyclists. These groups usually consist of individuals with varying degrees of fitness abilities. There is sure to be someone you will click with in the group. Or if you belong to a health club, post an ISO (in search of) on the bulletin board. You can also speak to some of the trainers on the floor. They might have clients who would love to partner train. You may even find someone to share personal training sessions, which is an excellent way to make them more affordable.

If you've been struggling to remain consistent with your workouts, Tip #28 is an especially effective strategy to employ. Begin right now by giving some thought on a potential exercise buddy. Once you come up with a friend or family member who may appreciate the "buddy system" and share your commitment, go ahead. **Contact him or her and make a plan!**

FOOD FOR THOUGHT... QUESTIONS & REFLECTIONS

1. What has been your experience exercising with a buddy? Do you feel like your personality is better suited for partner or solo workouts?

   _____

   _____

   _____

   _____

   _____

2. What types of exercises can you envision yourself regularly participating in with a partner?

   _____

   _____

   _____

   _____

   _____

3. What do you believe might be the advantages of partner workouts?

_____
_____
_____
_____
_____
_____

ACTION STEPS & EXERCISES

1. Think about friends or family members who might like to begin exercising with you. Contact those individuals and, if they're amenable, schedule a date for a workout session together.

2. If you don't know anyone who would be interested in the "buddy system," put your feelers out for a potential partner. Reach out by word of mouth or online.

3. What type of group sport/exercise activities might you find appealing? (Refer to the Action Steps of Tip #27.) Commit to attending a session and reach out to one or two individuals to whom you feel a connection. Be brave and broach the idea of scheduling a time to meet outside of the group sessions to try a workout together.

TIP #29

Tag exercise with another activity you enjoy: listening to music, reading, watching TV, or walking your dog.

Tip #27 centered upon joining an exercise class and how the camaraderie of a teacher and classmates, music, and prepayment can boost your motivation and increase your adherence to regular exercise.

In a similar vein, Tip #28—exercise with a buddy—fits

into the general scheme of Tip #29, adding enthusiasm by partnering up for workouts. A partner (especially a friend or family member) makes working out so much more enjoyable. You can catch up on the latest gossip, cheer each other on, or even partake in some friendly competition. Recently, a beautiful walking track was built around the local park in my town. Occasionally, I've been meeting my girlfriend and walking the path together with our dogs. Now, there's camaraderie and fun. What an incentive!

However, not everyone wants to participate in a class workout or with another person. For many individuals, especially beginners, exercising with others can feel intimidating or uncomfortable.

In general, I happen to be much more of a solo exerciser. My schedule changes so frequently that it's difficult to commit to a set time and place to work out. Plus I would rather not spend the extra time commuting to a studio. I'm fortunate enough to be a work-at-home professional with a small gym in my basement, so it's much more practical for me to hop on my treadmill or elliptical to exercise when I get a break. Although I love a motivational exercise class when I'm away on vacation or working out with my daughter when she's home for a visit, I primarily work out alone.

Nonetheless, if you decide that classes or a training buddy isn't for you, or at least not now, how can you make exercising more attractive and gratifying? It's an important question because when activities are fun and enjoyable, you'll be more likely to participate in them more often.

It can be considerably harder to exercise by yourself for 30–45 minutes without any external stimulation or motivation, right? So why not "tag" your favorite music or a great audiobook to listen to (through speakers or on headphones) with your workout? One of my clients was struggling to maintain consistency in her walking program. Once she started listening to books by her favorite mystery author on tape, she began to look forward to exercising. The anticipation of the next plot twist became an incentive for her to walk again and again. Sometimes, this client found that she had worked out for longer periods than planned because she had become wrapped up in the story. Similarly, if you're using a stationary bike, reading from a tablet or even an old-fashioned print book can make your workout time fly by.

Plenty of health clubs place their cardio machines in front of huge TVs, and most newer devices come equipped with individual TVs and computerized screens. If you own home equipment, situate it in a spot where you can easily see and hear the TV. Why not indulge in some guilty pleasure, like reality TV or sitcoms, while stepping or pedaling? Both of my exercise machines have stands where I can securely place my iPad. I love watching inspirational videos or listening to podcasts while I work out. On the other hand, my husband catches up on all of his favorite Netflix movies and shows when he works out at home.

While I've covered just a smidgen of activities you can pair with your exercise sessions, the choices run the gamut. Tap into your power of imagination, or solicit ideas from friends and family, as to what activities you can tag your exercise sessions with to make working out more alluring and gratifying.

FOOD FOR THOUGHT... QUESTIONS & REFLECTIONS

1. What thoughts come up for you when you imagine exercising alone and without any distractions (e.g. TV, music, talking on the phone, etc.)?

   _____
   _____
   _____
   _____
   _____
   _____

2. What activities might you tag to your exercise sessions to make them more enjoyable and make the time go by quickly?

   _____
   _____
   _____
   _____

ACTION STEPS & EXERCISES

1. Reflect on all the types of activities you enjoy and find gratifying that might tag nicely with exercise.

2. This week, experiment with tagging some of these activities to your typical workouts.

3. Note whether tagging activities to exercise increases your enjoyment, duration, intensity, and/or consistency of your workouts.

TIP #30

Increase daily movement whenever possible.

When I speak with folks about weight loss, inevitably there are a few people who swear they have a slow metabolism. It seems that, no matter what they do, they can't lose weight. Or if they do lose weight, it's at such a snail's pace that they become discouraged and disheartened. In the worst case scenarios, they give up, continuing to envy those individuals they believe to be the "lucky ones" who have a healthy or speedy metabolism.

It's true that some individuals do have endocrine disorders that can slow metabolism and make calorie burning and weight loss more difficult. However, the majority of people don't have metabolic problems. Rather, they have movement problems. That is, they're just not employing enough—or the best—tactics to yield significant weight loss results.

If despite working out on a regular basis and watching your calorie intake, you still feel that the rate of your weight loss is slower than you would expect, or you still struggle to maintain your ideal weight, don't be so quick to blame it on a sluggish metabolism.

By all means, discuss your health concerns with a physician. Your doctor can take a metabolic profile, and any worry you have may be quickly alleviated if your blood work results are normal and your hormone levels lie within a healthy range. If it turns out that you do have a hormonal imbalance, there are usually ways to correct an excess or deficit so that your body can do what it's designed to do in order to function properly. Nonetheless, if your lab results indicate that your hormones are balanced and you are otherwise healthy, it's time to look at another reason weight loss might be such a challenge for you—that is, lack of enough movement during your day.

Because when it comes to weight reduction or gain, for the most part, we're playing a numbers game. Too much food consumption and not enough energy expenditure will cause you to gain weight. Eat less and move more, and you will lose weight. Although this may be an oversimplified explanation, fundamentally, it illustrates how the energy equation works.

Your BMR (Basal Metabolic Rate) is the energy required for you to live, the energy needed for you to breathe, your heart to beat, your blood to circulate, and even your eyelids to flutter. Thermogenesis, or the thermic effect of food (TEF), is the amount of energy expenditure above the resting metabolic rate, due to the cost of processing food for use and storage. (Yes, even the process of digestion burns calories.) Your daily caloric requirement is determined by your BMR, TEF, and what is referred to as NEAT (Non-Exercise Activity Thermogenesis) or NEPA (Non-Exercise Physical Activity). NEAT or NEPA is the energy expended for everything we do that is not sleeping, eating, or sports-like exercise. It ranges from the energy spent walking to work, typing, performing yard work, housekeeping, and even fidgeting. NEAT or NEPA is a significant part of the energy equation. Although NEPA and NEAT are often used interchangeably, for simplicity's sake, I will use NEAT when referring to the energy required for non-exercise activity during a day.

Your BMR accounts for approximately 60 percent of your daily caloric needs. The thermic effect of food accounts for about 10–15 percent of your energy requirements. The remainder of your energy requirements is dependent upon how active you are during both intentional exercise and NEAT activities. The latter includes typical life activities, like cleaning, shopping, walking, etc. NEAT can account for as little as 15 percent of energy expenditure in very sedentary individuals and up to 50 percent in very active individuals.

Researchers have performed experiments to uncover what occurs inside the human body that determines whether one stores excess food as fat or utilizes (caloric burn) it for fuel. What is the difference regarding those processes? The subjects who burned fat off naturally increased their NEAT, while those who added fat did not! Again, understand that NEAT is all of the calories you burn through simple activities of daily life—like twiddling your thumbs, tapping your feet, chewing gum, cooking, shopping at the grocery store, etc. NEAT accounts for HUNDREDS of calories burned each day, which is significantly more than most people burn in the gym!

So, what does all of this mean? You can increase your NEAT, *and* it will make a difference in terms of weight loss. Think about your average day. If you were going to make a deliberate effort to increase NEAT, what might you do? Perhaps, instead of sitting down, hold walking meetings with coworkers, or talk on the phone using a headset while moving around your workplace. Set a timer to go off every hour to remind you to stand, stretch, or get up for a drink of water. And how about the many ideas you have often heard (including some I suggested in past chapters)? For example, park the car farther away from the entrance to a building, take stairs rather than elevators and escalators, or get off the bus or train one stop early. Choosing any or all of these options will indeed make a difference when it comes to reaching your weight loss goals. Because, as I often repeat, small changes lead to huge results.

I hope that now you're excited and have begun to think about how you can increase your NEAT. (*Wouldn't it be neat to boost your NEAT?*) You never know, maybe you can start a movement to inspire others. Literally a movement to move more often!

FOOD FOR THOUGHT... QUESTIONS & REFLECTIONS

1. What types of activities—aside from regularly scheduled workout sessions—do you typically perform daily?

___

Weekly?

___

2. What strategies can you employ to increase your activity level during your day?

_____
_____
_____
_____
_____
_____
_____
_____
_____
_____

3. In the past, have you believed your metabolism was slow, normal, or fast? After reading the information above, has your opinion changed?

_____
_____
_____

ACTION STEPS & EXERCISES

1. Make a list of actions you can take (like those suggested above and more) to increase your daily NEAT.

_____
_____
_____
_____
_____
_____
_____
_____
_____
_____
_____
_____
_____

2. Set alerts on your phone or computer to remind you to get up and move every hour.

3. Consider purchasing a fitness tracker to count your daily steps. Set a goal to increase your steps on a weekly basis.

4. If you are still struggling to lose weight despite your best efforts and fear you might have a slow metabolism, schedule an appointment with your physician for a check-up and to have a metabolic profile taken.

TIP #31

Wear a pedometer every day.

You're already aware that, although what you eat has the greatest impact on the number on the scale, exercise and staying physically active are essential components when it comes to weight control.

Unfortunately, we live relatively sedentary lives. Even if we include regular visits to the gym, for most of us, the rest of our days are spent sitting at the computer, commuting in cars, or watching TV while relaxing on the couch.

Tip #30 talked about the importance of NEAT (Non-Exercise Activity Thermogenesis). Which means you now understand that maintaining a healthy body weight or losing weight depends on burning more calories than we consume. So any way we can introduce extra movement into our daily lives is going to help. And there is no easier method to boost daily movement than by increasing the number of steps we take each day, that is by walking, running, or climbing stairs.

A pedometer is a portable device that measures your physical activity level, primarily the number of steps you take throughout the day. Unless you have tracked steps using a pedometer, you probably have no idea how many, or how few, steps you take daily. The answer may surprise you.

Wearing a pedometer is an excellent means of heightening your awareness of how much you do—or don't—move, and it can be a great motivator to get you up on your feet. When I wear my pedometer, if I notice a low count in the afternoon, I feel much more inspired to take a break from my desk and take the dog for a loop around the block.

Pedometers are inexpensive, convenient, and user-friendly. You may even own one and not realize it. If you have a smartphone, such as the iPhone or Samsung Galaxy, it already has a built-in step counter. Plus you can download a multitude of apps that will count your steps for you. The only problem with that strategy is that you will not get an accurate total unless that phone is turned on and with you every time you start moving. If you purchase a pedometer, however, you would wear it on your belt or the waistband of your clothing. A pedometer is small and lightweight. You can then have it with you all the time.

If you love technology, there are hi-tech trackers, such as Fitbit or Jawbone, that will also monitor your heart rate, estimate the number of calories you burn, and even your sleep quantity and quality. But you don't necessarily need that extra information. Simply tracking your steps with an easy-to-use, inexpensive pedometer has been proven to be highly motivating, fun, and therefore beneficial.

Studies have shown that using a pedometer increases physical activity by at least 1,800 to 4,500 steps a day, which is equivalent to walking an extra one to two and a quarter miles. Enlist a buddy, and you can get a friendly competition going—see who can "score" more steps each day.

The majority of health organizations recommend that we accumulate at least 10,000 steps per day. On average, 2,000 steps equals approximately one mile, so walking 10,000 steps equates to walking about five miles. Although that is a great goal to strive for, remember that *it's just one part of a holistic approach* to remaining healthy and managing weight. If you're extremely sedentary—clocking in at only 2,000–3,000 steps per day—but you eat a relatively healthy diet *and then* increase your daily steps to 10,000, you just might drop a few pounds or have an easier time maintaining a healthy weight. Nevertheless, if you incorporate those additional steps with the mindset that you can then treat yourself to French fries at lunch, those extra steps will not create a "balance" between your exercise and your non-nutritious, high-caloric intake.

Whichever road you choose (no pun intended), tracking your steps—in particular, with the help of a pedometer—can help you increase your daily movement. **Aim to increase the number of steps you take by 500–1,000 steps per week.** Introduce some creativity into this exercise (pun intended!). Take stairs rather than the elevator, go to the work restroom on a different floor, or walk into the bank rather than using the drive-through teller. Before you know it, you'll average 10,000 steps a day! Go ahead, then, and purchase that pedometer. Wear it daily and watch as motivation steps up and the pounds step down!

FOOD FOR THOUGHT... QUESTIONS & REFLECTIONS

1. How many steps do you think you average on most days of the week? What are your thoughts when you contemplate using a pedometer?

   _____
   _____
   _____
   _____

2. In what ways do you typically "measure" your movement and/or steps?

   _____
   _____

3. List any ideas you have on when and where you might increase your steps during your typical day.

   _____
   _____
   _____

_____

_____

_____

_____

ACTION STEPS & EXERCISES

1. Buy that pedometer. See Appendix C for suggestions of brands.

2. Wear your new pedometer daily and get used to tracking your steps. After seven days, determine your daily average.

3. Start with a goal of increasing your average daily steps by 500 more each week. Gradually increase the number of steps you walk or run as you continuously extend your goal. Reaching 10,000 steps/day becomes your ultimate objective.

4. Add accountability by inviting a friend to wear a pedometer and track his or her steps too. Compare your counts daily or weekly.

5. Journal or chart the number of steps you take per day when using the pedometer to gauge your progress—inspire yourself that way!

TIP #32

Check serving sizes on foods' labels. Do the math in order to keep portion sizes and consumption in line with your weight loss goals.

If you've ever attempted to lose weight by following a set diet plan, you know that significant components are awareness of, and adherence to, portion sizes. It's for this reason that dieters are instructed to measure the weight of foods, count out the number of pieces in a serving size of packaged foods, or count points and add up calories during the course of a day or week. Even if you're eating the healthiest of foods imaginable, if you consume too much of them, you will effectively sabotage your weight loss efforts.

Based on the title of this book, you can reasonably assume that I'm not a huge advocate of starting a diet, and you would be right. Rather than "going on a diet," I want to help you tweak your eating and activity habits so that you create a new lifestyle that supports losing weight and maintaining a target weight or weight range. Nonetheless, that doesn't mean you don't need to pay attention to serving sizes and portion control. Checking labels and appropriately adjusting your intake is part of the new, healthy lifestyle routines you will want to establish.

Nowhere does the concept of portion size become more confusing than when purchasing packaged foods. Manufacturers are notorious for duping us into thinking that a particular foodstuff is a great low-calorie option when it's not. The same holds true for low-fat, low-sodium, low-cholesterol, or any other labeling that might influence what you choose to purchase. Food manufacturers are in the business of making money, and they really aren't concerned about whether or not you gain weight in the process. If they can convince you that their product is a healthier or lower-calorie option than another, purchases increase and so do their revenues.

However, learning to be an educated consumer is relatively easy. By doing so, you can become more aware of marketing tricks, "do the math," and make better choices. Allow me to provide an example and some insight.

I love Amy's Organic Soups (www.amys.com/our-foods?onthemenu%5B0%5D=soups). I keep several cans in my pantry at all times. Like many other people, when I look at the soup can, it appears to be a single serving. However, when I examine the nutritional label, I notice that a serving size is one cup and that there are two cups per can. Each serving of this particular soup contains 150 calories. When I do the math, I can easily determine that consuming the entire can equates to ingesting 300 calories. Now, that can make for a nutritious lunch if I add in a few whole grain crackers and maybe some salad or fruit. Opting for that route, I'll probably end up with a pretty healthy 400–450-calorie meal. However, if a can of soup and salad are not enough to satisfy me, and I decide to eat a sandwich as well, I'll need to rethink eating the entire can's worth. Considering most sandwiches will total approximately 350–400 calories, when I add a full can of soup, my meal becomes 650–700 calories; an excessive amount of food and calories for one meal. So if I want that sandwich too, I better stick to half of the can for 150 calories or only half a sandwich.

Sometimes, especially during cold winter months, I have soup as a late afternoon snack. One cup (one-half of a can) is a perfect portion; but if I were to have the entire can, I would be taking in too many calories at snack time to maintain my healthy weight range over the long haul. Once in a great while won't make that much of a difference. However, if I consistently eat the entire can of soup at lunch time, along with a full sandwich, and another entire can of soup when I choose that as an afternoon snack, those excess calories will begin to add up. My scale will probably alert me that I'm not paying attention to portion size (and the information on labels) as much as I—or anyone else—should.

The next time you're in the supermarket, just for fun, pull out some of the prepackaged dinners in the freezer section. Many, even those that are supposedly "healthy" actually indicate that there are two servings per package (likely in smaller print). So if you don't look closely at the package—and in particular, the nutrition label—you might believe that you would be purchasing an individual-sized meal, yet you would actually be buying enough for two people. Note too that a single serving is probably not going to satisfy your appetite sufficiently.

Some of the worst offenders are the small, allegedly individual-sized snack foods like chips or pretzels. Take a look at the calorie count of those products, and you may think, "Hey, this isn't too bad or unhealthy—it's only 100 calories. I can enjoy these with my lunch or as a snack." Examine the serving size a little more closely, though. You'll see that some brands will list two or even two and one-half servings per bag. Start multiplying calories by serving size, and you will quickly realize "not so bad" is really "not so good."

Be cautious with foods that are packaged in larger bags, such as nuts or dried fruits. And some foods will list a serving size in ounces or tea-/tablespoons. In order to stick to an appropriate amount, you'll need to read each label carefully and measure out the proper weight or quantity.

The lesson to be learned from Tip #32 is simple: **If you pay attention and adhere to portion sizes, you'll further your efforts to alter your habits and lose weight...without going on a diet.** This is just another of my many strategies that will ease your weight reduction efforts and lead you to your ultimate goal.

FOOD FOR THOUGHT... QUESTIONS & REFLECTIONS

1. What has been your experience with reading food labels? How often are you in the habit of doing so, and what information do you usually check?

   _____
   _____
   _____
   _____
   _____
   _____

2. In what ways do you typically attempt to monitor portion control?

   _____
   _____
   _____
   _____
   _____

ACTION STEPS & EXERCISES

1. Purchase a food scale if you don't already own one. (See Appendix C for suggested types.)

2. Make sure you have measuring cups and spoons handy in your kitchen and begin using them to control your portions.

3. Read all of the nutrition labels, including—and particularly—serving sizes on the foods in your home.

4. Next time you're at the grocery store, check the serving size and calorie total for the foods you regularly purchase or any new ones you're thinking about trying.

5. Think about your entire meal and how many total calories you want to consume. Write down any instance in which you feel you need to adjust portion size compared to your habits of the past.

_____

_____

_____

_____

_____

6. Practice doling out the portion sizes that will remain within your chosen parameters—meaning those that will support your weight loss efforts, not to mention your overall health.

TIP #33

Use measuring cups and spoons as serving utensils.

I've been serving meals and snacks using measuring cups and measuring spoons as utensils for years. It has helped both my family and me to become conscious of how much a serving size is and what a proper portion looks like. Have you ever considered this strategy?

In Tip #32, we called attention to the benefit of reading food labels and understanding serving sizes and portion control. Next, we will take that concept a bit further and discuss how we can apply it at home every day.

I'm suggesting that you use measuring cups and spoons as serving utensils. Now, I can imagine your thought process. "Ellen, you told me I could lose weight without going on a diet or counting and measuring every little thing I eat." And yes, I do believe that. On the other hand, you still have to understand what a portion size looks (and feels) like (for example, one cup of rice or cereal). Whether we want to accept it or not, weight loss and maintenance do depend on the number of calories we eat. And anyone who says calories don't matter does not understand energy balance.

That being said, Tip #33 is meant to guide you toward educating yourself and being mindful when serving foods and snacks to yourself and your family. Even when you're eating the healthiest of fare, as I've described before, if you are not paying attention to proper serving size, you will probably consume more than you need in order to meet your energy demands each day (remember, food is fuel). Consistently bringing in too much fuel—too many calories, no matter what source of food they are coming from—will increase your chances of gaining weight.

I recommend, then, that you buy several inexpensive sets of measuring cups and spoons. The next time you're ready to serve your family pasta, rice, mashed potatoes, applesauce, or even ice cream, check the serving size on the label and use the proper sized measuring cup to dish out the food. You can use the same trick for spreads and condiments, like salad dressings, hummus, and peanut butter—basically, any fare that is easy to overeat if you're not paying attention to calories per serving size. If there is a particular food you reach for frequently, like a breakfast cereal, you can even leave the measuring cup in the box to use as a scooper.

Very soon, you'll be able to identify what a proper serving is, even without measuring it. So rather than do away with a favorite food such as pasta or mashed potatoes, try instead to stick to an appropriate portion size, and calculate it within your daily calorie allotment.

By implementing Tip #33, you'll also begin to recognize how oversized the portions are at restaurants, which will remind you to bring half of your meal home or share it with a dining partner. Couple this practice with slowing down when you eat and pausing before diving in for seconds, and you will train your body and mind to become conscious of when you're satiated. You'll discover that a serving size of grains, pasta, or potatoes, along with an adequate helping of protein, is actually enough to satisfy you. And you will find yourself enjoying favorite foods while consuming reasonable—rather than excessive—portions. Once you introduce this kind of concentrated attention to your eating habits, it's possible, if not probable, that you will lose weight. And you'd be doing it without having the need to go on a strict diet plan.

Intriguing? Commit to Tip #33, allow some time to put it to the test, and realize the results in weight loss and well-being!

FOOD FOR THOUGHT...
QUESTIONS & REFLECTIONS

1. How often do you turn your attention to portion size when serving food at home?

   _____

   _____

2. What methods have you used to dish out foods at meal time or when eating snacks?

   _____

   _____

   _____

3. What are your thoughts when you consider the idea of using measuring cups and spoons as serving utensils?

   _____

   _____

   _____

   _____

ACTION STEPS & EXERCISES

1. Purchase a few sets of low-cost measuring cups and spoons.

2. Take a careful look at the labels on the foods you have at home that you regularly consume, and note the serving size on each. At your next meal or snack, measure the appropriate "one portion" and eat (or drink) it. Resist going back for seconds.

3. After you finish that meal or snack, reflect on how you feel emotionally and physically. Are you satiated?

4. Give your body a few weeks to adjust to eating smaller portions, and then check in to see if this strategy has helped you to take off a few pounds.

TIP #34

Do not serve family style, except when it comes to salads, veggies, or fresh fruit.

Take the old expression, "Out of sight, out of mind," and flip it (look at the converse). You will get "in sight, top of the mind." You now have two truths regarding food and eating habits. Don't you find that, the moment you see food you enjoy, it causes a strong desire to eat it right then and there? When coveted fare is in front of us—be it, for example, in our refrigerators, in advertisements, or even on a coworker's desk—our brains instantly connect to the "pleasure zone." In other words, the sight of that sumptuous food automatically brings to mind how delicious it will taste and how good we will feel when we eat it!

Sight plays a significant role in our enjoyment of food. When we serve ourselves, we would be wise to consider that. When it's time to sit down for a meal, having a single plate filled with proper serving sizes of nutritious and delicious fare makes good sense. However, if there's an abundance of that food available in plain sight—which is what happens when food is served family style—we'll probably have great difficulty with keeping to appropriate serving sizes. Those edibles look, smell, and taste delectable, so as long as there are more of them in front of us, we'll be tempted to dig in again and again.

Too many people are in the habit of dining "family style." Perhaps we reside in homes where the cook serves meals in this manner—placing platters or baking dishes filled with the night's preparations directly in front of us on the kitchen table, along with large serving utensils. We may visit the homes of friends and relatives who serve meals similarly. Or we frequent family style restaurants. The invitation is clear: Take as much food as you want and refill your plate as often as you would like.

The problem this scenario creates is that it becomes easy to overeat. There are plenty of times when we aren't in control of serving style, but when it comes to the meals we serve in our homes, we can and should be accountable. And that's why I recommend that you avoid serving meals family style at home.

Certainly, this can be a hard habit to break, but it is indeed possible and well worth the effort. Eating from family style served meals is a mindless invitation to overeat. Even if you believe that you don't eat in excess or indulge in seconds too often, I'll bet that, if measured, the amount of food scooped onto your plate has you consuming unnecessary calories. When weight reduction is a priority, this change in serving style can surely help eliminate some of the excess calories you may not realize are sneaking into your daily intake.

Why not take the few small steps that will remove any inadvertent enticement to overeat? Rather than placing serving platters and pans on the dining table, instead plate each dish with a single serving of food before putting it on the table. Hold the reasons you want to lose weight at the forefront of your mind. Those are your reminders of how valuable a modicum of extra effort can be. And this will be especially the case if your new approach proves to be an effective tool!

But what happens if you are not the person in charge of serving the family meals? Then it's time for some communication. Ask for the support you need while on your weight loss journey. Discuss with that individual why you want to make this switch in serving style. Maybe you can offer to dish out the food onto everyone's plates. I'm sure the help will be appreciated. Then, if you want seconds, you'll need to physically get up from the table and head to the stove or counter to get more. That fact alone may curb the habit of reaching for seconds when you are, in truth, no longer hungry. Look at another bright side—in changing your meal serving practice, you'll potentially wind up with leftovers for lunch the next day!

Keep in mind there is an exception to this general rule—that is when it comes to meals that include salad, vegetables, or fruit. Some dishes served family style can work perfectly well within a healthy food plan. As long as those salads or vegetables aren't swimming in sauces, butter, oil, or any other high-fat, high-calorie ingredients. The same holds true for fresh fruit desserts. In fact, I encourage you to leave that type of wholesome fare on the table. These are the kinds of nourishing foods that fill you up and are comparatively lower in calories relative to volume and nutritional value. Set those veggies and fresh fruits right on the table and indulge! Go ahead and relish second servings of those selections as much as you would like!

FOOD FOR THOUGHT...
QUESTIONS & REFLECTIONS

1. How do you typically serve meals in your home?

   _____

   _____

   _____

2. How often do you eat at family style restaurants?

   _____

3. Reflect on the advantages to no longer serving family style or frequenting restaurants that do so.

   _____

   _____

   _____

   _____

   _____

   _____

4. If you're used to eating family style meals, and decide that a shift in habit will benefit you (and your family), who would you need to discuss this change with?

_____

_____

_____

_____

_____

_____

ACTION STEPS & EXERCISES

1. Choose a convenient time to discuss the upcoming modification of your serving style with anyone in your household who might be impacted, and have the conversation.

2. Commit to a date to begin implementing your new approach to serving meals.

3. Take note of each meal's menu—which items you will refrain from putting on the table vs which fare you can place on the table. (Those healthy vegetables and fresh fruits!)

4. The next time you're dining and begin to think about taking a second helping, be mindful and pause before you act. Ask yourself, "Am I still hungry or just in the habit of taking seconds?" Respond by acting in line with your answer.

5. At the completion of your meal, take a few minutes to contemplate how you feel physically and emotionally.

TIP #35

Get seven to eight hours of sleep every night.

I believe so strongly—and often tell my clients—that when it comes to weight loss, "*Fatigue is the enemy.*" It turns out that research backs me up on this assertion. Getting seven to eight hours of sleep most nights of the week is critical for losing and maintaining a healthy weight.

In fact, I can provide you with five solid reasons why this contention holds true:

The sleep-deprived brain sets us up for making poor choices. The prefrontal cortex (PFC) is the part of the brain responsible for rational, analytical thinking, problem-solving, making sensible decisions, and impulse control. When we're sleep deprived, the PFC can't function optimally; it's as if the lights are dimmed in that part of our brains. But the lights go on full force in our limbic—emotional—brain center. When we're overly tired, the amygdala—the part of our brain that processes emotions—takes over. In other words, we react with our feelings rather than with logic. The result is that we are overly emotional *and* lack impulse control when exhausted. Therefore, that part of our brains searches for anything that will temporarily make us feel better, calm us down, or give us instant energy. So, we end up buying a candy bar from the vending machine at 3:00 p.m. rather than eating the apple and nuts we brought from home. Or we choose the bacon cheeseburger at dinner rather than the salmon and salad. Now you can understand that when the limbic brain is in charge, which it tends to be when you are chronically sleep-deprived, willpower goes out the door. Effectively, your weight loss goals become less of a priority during those moments.

When we're sleep-deprived, we tend to exercise less intensely and less frequently. When we're exhausted, it's next to impossible to force ourselves to work out or even go for a walk. We'll hit the snooze button despite our best intentions to get to the gym in the morning. We'll tell ourselves, "It's OK. I'll put off exercise until the end of the day," but later decide that we're just too darn tired. Night after sleepless night turns into day after day of missed workouts. Now, that is certainly not a very good formula for accelerating weight loss and maintenance plans. Don't you agree?

Staying up late at night often leads to consumption of excess calories; and most of the time, those calories are derived from the non-nutritious fare that, in turn, precipitates weight gain. A study in the American Journal of Clinical Nutrition found that when subjects were starved of sleep, late-night snacking increased, and the subjects were more likely to choose high-carbohydrate foods. Numerous studies indicate that lack of sleep leads to increased cravings for energy-dense, high-carbohydrate foods. So a tired brain appears to crave junk food *and* lacks the impulse control to say "No!"

Sleep deprivation wreaks havoc on our hormones. The appetite hormone, ghrelin, signals to the brain when it's time to eat. Leptin is another hormone which tells us when we're satiated. Chronic sleep deprivation has been shown to increase production of ghrelin, while leptin production plummets, thereby directing your brain to sound the alarm; you want to eat more. And if that's not enough, there is a cortisol spike that comes from a deficit of sleep. This stress hormone signals the brain to conserve energy to fuel us during waking hours. Our bodies, then, become more apt to retain fat.

Last but not least, sleep deprivation alters our metabolism (and not in a good way). One study from the University of Chicago revealed that within only four days of insufficient sleep, the body's ability to process insulin—a hormone needed to transform sugar, starches, and other foods into energy—goes awry. The researchers found that insulin sensitivity (the cell's ability to utilize insulin properly) decreased by more than 30 percent. Here is where the problem arises: When the body doesn't respond appropriately to insulin, it becomes difficult to process glucose in the bloodstream, so it ends up being stored as fat. The lesson to be learned here is that inadequate sleep hampers one's metabolism and thus hinders weight loss or, even worse, causes weight gain.

The following is a recap of the five reasons why you should be sure to get at least seven to eight hours of sleep as often as possible.

You can't reason or focus clearly and make favorable food choices when you're tired.

You'll end up skipping too many exercise sessions.

You'll consume an excess of non-nutritious, high-calorie junk food late at night when you should otherwise be asleep.

You'll disrupt the hormonal processes that regulate appetite and fat burning.

You'll impair your metabolism, thereby decreasing insulin sensitivity and increasing fat storage.

If you're still struggling to lose weight despite having made positive changes regarding your eating and movement habits, turn your attention to sleep. I recommend that you start by performing a "self-check"—track the time you get to bed and wake up each morning for a week or so. Determine how many hours of sleep you average per night. If that number falls below seven, start setting goals focused on going to bed at a time that will allow for at least seven hours of sleep. Only turn your attention back to your daily eating habits once you've cultivated new bedtime habits. At the root of Tip #35 is this research-based theory: **An increase in sleep may amount to a decrease in pounds.** Why not put it to the test? You can become lighter in body and mind.

FOOD FOR THOUGHT... QUESTIONS & REFLECTIONS

1. In what ways have you noticed fatigue impacts your food choices and decisions?

   _____
   _____
   _____
   _____
   _____
   _____
   _____

2. How many hours of sleep do you believe you get each night?

   _____

3. How rested and refreshed do you feel on most mornings?

   _____
   _____
   _____

4. If you usually sleep less than seven or eight hours per night, what daytime or nighttime habits would you need to shift in order to increase the amount of time you sleep?

_____

_____

_____

_____

_____

_____

_____

_____

ACTION STEPS & EXERCISES

1. Self-check: Track the number of hours of sleep you get each night for a week. How many hours of sleep did you average?

2. Create SMART Goals around the behaviors you're willing to change in order to get seven to eight hours of sleep each night. (See Appendix D for guidelines to create SMART Goals.)

3. If you find it difficult to fall asleep, speak with your doctor or research the many strategies you can employ to fall asleep easier. (Of the many, here are some examples: muscle relaxation exercises, deep breathing or meditation, listening to low-volume, soothing sounds or music, and refraining from the use of your mobile phone or TV for at least one hour before bedtime.)

TIP #36

Wear form-fitting clothing.

There is a common belief I've noticed amongst individuals who are working on weight loss that, until you reach goal weight, loose and baggy clothing looks and feels better. Ask any stylist and you might be surprised to learn that form-fitting apparel makes you look thinner; that is, as long as it is properly sized. Although you might feel a bit more body conscious in tailored outfits, they should not feel uncomfortable or tight.

Nevertheless, one of the major benefits of spending

your days in more restrictive clothing is that you *will* notice right away when your weight is creeping up. Your garments will begin to feel snug, and that awareness will spur you to start paying closer attention to note if your new healthy habits are sliding. By the same token, when you're losing weight, you'll find joy in slipping into your clothing and realizing it feels and looks a bit loose. And, others will notice as well. However, no matter what body size you're currently at, well-fitting tailored clothing is way more attractive than shapeless, baggy apparel.

Let me share a story with you. Recently, when coaching a client who had just achieved a milestone, having lost 40 pounds, I noted a lack of enthusiasm in her voice. I thought she would be jumping for joy. When I questioned the disappointment I sensed in her voice she replied, "I went to a party this past weekend. A lot of folks I hadn't seen in several weeks were there. I was expecting everyone to see how much thinner I was, but not a single one said it looked like I had lost weight." I can empathize with how discouraging this was for her, because most of us hope that our hard work and efforts will be acknowledged.

So I asked about what she wore to the event, "Did you buy a new outfit for the party or wear something that hadn't fit you in years?" There was a moment of silence on the other end of the phone before she replied, "No, I wore what I always wear to parties. My black, silky palazzo pants and a loose-fitting top that matches. I dress it up with jewelry." Essentially, my client had worn relatively shapeless clothing; not a more tapered outfit that might show off the curves of her body. How would anyone notice her transformation? Especially for this particular client who, in the past, had always prided herself on "being able to hide her excess weight" by wearing loose clothing with elastic waist-bands and flowing materials as well as avoiding clingy or tight-fitting garments.

There are several problems inherent in my client's (and so many other individuals') thought process. For starters, when you regularly wear loose clothing, it is hard to detect a difference in weight changes in either direction. Without the message from your pants, skirts, or belts getting tighter, you may not notice your weight is creeping up. Similarly, you will not note the changes in your body regarding a decrease in weight if you can't tell that your clothes look and feel looser. Aside from the reading on the scale (which we know is a fickle friend that can fluctuate by several pounds on any given day), the way your clothing fits—or not—is a great GPS when your aim is weight reduction. Garment fit will let you know if your efforts are taking you in the right direction, or if you need to recalculate and redirect.

The second reason that wearing form-fitting clothing is to your advantage: No matter what size you are, form-fitting clothing will, believe it or not, help you come across as more attractive—in other words, you'll look nicer. I often recommend that clients meet with a professional image consultant or find a personal shopper with a great eye in their local department stores. Personal shoppers' services are often free for customers. Why ask an image consultant or personal shopper for advice? Because it provides you with the opportunity to discover many strategies and styles that will make you appear thinner. At the same time, you'll also see and hear for yourself that wearing baggy clothing is not one of them.

Last, but not least, the third reason it behooves you to wear more tailored attire is, as I touched upon above, snug, uncomfortable fitting clothing is one of the first signs that your weight reduction efforts have gone awry. I know how tempting it is to forgo stepping on the scale when you've lapsed somewhat along your journey. And how easy it is to rationalize that you will weigh in when you get back on track. If you're wearing loose, baggy clothing and avoiding the scale, a few gained pounds can quickly turn into many since you aren't utilizing a measurement tool. Well, in short, the feel of tight clothing can be highly motivating to step on the scale to check in, and then get you back on track.

When you lose (or have lost) a significant amount of weight, celebrate with some new, more form-fitting clothing that makes you look great. You may be thinking, "I don't want to spend money on new clothing until I'm at my goal weight." If so, first go shopping in your closet—you might very well find some lovely clothes that have not fit for a while but do now. Or buy just a few form fitting items. An excellent tailor will easily be able to take them in when you lose more weight and reach your target.

The message I hope you glean from Tip #36 is to **dress your best in more form-fitting, beautiful clothing, regardless of your current weight.** I promise, your friends and family will begin to notice how sharp and put-together you're looking, and the compliments will fly! Enjoy the adventure and remember that small changes (of clothing that is—wink, wink) will lead to great results.

FOOD FOR THOUGHT...
QUESTIONS & REFLECTIONS

1. How often do you reach for loose fitting clothing (such as leggings, sweat pants, baggy shirts, or dresses) vs more form-fitting clothing (such as jeans, zipper and button slacks or skirts, or tapered shirts or dresses)?

   _____

2. What percentage of clothing in your closet do you choose not to wear because you believe it's not appropriate for the size of your body right now?

   _____

3. On a scale of 1–10 (1=awful, 10=fabulous), how do you usually feel when getting dressed to go out for the day or special occasions? If you gave yourself a rating of 6 or below, what might you do to increase your positive feelings towards the way you dress?

   _____

   _____

   _____

   _____

ACTION STEPS & EXERCISES

1. Schedule a block of time to go through your closet. Pull out some pieces that you haven't worn in a while because they had gotten too tight. If you have already lost some weight, try them on once again.

2. If you can't find any clothing in your closet that feels good to wear, and you have the budget, make an appointment with a personal shopper at your favorite department store and buy a few form-fitting outfits.

3. Set aside a comfortable budget for "reward shopping" when you reach small milestones. For instance, buy a new outfit each time you lose five or ten pounds.

4. Buy one pair of great-fitting jeans or slacks. Commit to wearing them at least once a week. If you notice they're getting snug, pay close attention to your daily health habits. If they begin to feel loose, celebrate! Make sure you know the name and number of a good seamstress for alterations once they get too loose.

5. If you've lost some weight (even if you have not yet reached your goal or target range), spend some time with family and friends wearing your new clothing. Flaunt your fabulousness and accept any compliments you receive (without any, "But I have more weight to lose," or similar self-deprecating remarks). And pat yourself on the back too. You deserve it!

TIP #37

Cook healthy foods in advance and freeze in individual containers.

This tip needs little, if any, explanation. Cook healthy foods in advance, and freeze them in individual containers. It just makes good sense that whenever we spend time cooking, we can (and probably should) make enough for more than one meal. That way, we will have great choices available on the days we don't have time to prepare a home-cooked meal from scratch and one less day of pots and pans to clean!

All of us should recognize that to lose weight and keep it off, we need to get back into our kitchens and cook. It is decidedly easier to eat nutritiously when we are the ones controlling what ingredients go into a given dish. At the same time, however, we lead such busy lives that cooking every night is difficult. Discovering easier ways to prepare home-cooked meals in advance, then, will increase the frequency of our doing so. Right?

I figured out early on that it's much more feasible for me to cook on the weekends when I have more time available, feel less rushed and stressed, and can enjoy experimenting with new recipes and ingredients. As long as I'm spending time in the kitchen, I'm definitely going to make sure there's enough food prepared for several meals.

That being said, we need to plan and prep before we head into the kitchen. If we're going to double or even triple a single recipe, we must purchase that much more of each ingredient when we go to the market. We have to ensure that our shopping lists take that into account.

We also need pots, pans, and casserole dishes that will accommodate larger portions. And we definitely ought to have quality freezer containers on hand. Personally, I like glass containers with lids. Aside from freezing in them, I can use them to reheat meals in the oven or, when rushed, in the microwave. (The latter is especially convenient when I forget to take out food to defrost in the morning—which I admit I do at times.) I purchased from Amazon, an extremely reasonably-priced set of glass containers with airtight lids—plus enough size options to freeze foods for one, two, or more meals. And let's not forget freezer tape. (Did you know there was such a thing?) That way, we can label and date the contents so we know what's inside. Here's another trick: Write not only the dish and the date you prepared it, but also whether there is enough servings to feed one, two, or even a greater number of people.

So if you're ready to give this strategy a try, here's a road map to follow: First, choose a few recipes that intrigue you, keeping in mind that stews, soups, casseroles, and dishes with sauces freeze best. Next, make a list of the ingredients for your dishes of choice and multiply the quantities of those ingredients, based on how much you plan to cook. If you don't already have them, invest in larger, well-manufactured pots, pans, and casserole dishes. One of my favorite cooking tools is a crock pot. I can prepare meals in advance, place all of the ingredients in it that morning and have a delicious and fragrant dish ready in time for dinner. My crock pot is large enough so that there are always leftovers to freeze in individual containers. If you don't already own one, consider the three-in-one cooking system by Ninja. This product can be used for browning, sautéing, baking, and as a crock pot. Check out my product suggestions in Appendix C.

Ready to get cooking? Once you find a time slot in your week that suits you, you are set to go. Play your favorite background music and have fun cooking for not only one, but several meals to come!

FOOD FOR THOUGHT... QUESTIONS & REFLECTIONS

1. What do you think about cooking for more than one meal? Does it seem like an excellent idea, or overwhelming and just "too much"? If this concept seems daunting, what might you do to make it easier and more enjoyable to give this strategy a try?

_____

_____

_____

_____

_____

_____

_____

_____

_____

_____

2. Based on your schedule, what day(s) are best for to prepare a few dishes that you can freeze for future meals?

_____

_____

_____

_____

3. Do you have quality cookware and storage containers? What might you need to purchase so that you are prepared to batch cook meals for freezing?

_____

_____

_____

_____

_____

_____

_____

ACTION STEPS & EXERCISES

1. Review your schedule for this upcoming week. Choose one time slot in which you can commit to cooking a healthy meal. Mark it on your calendar.

2. Choose a recipe that excites you. Decide if you'll double or triple the recipe. Multiply and add enough ingredients to your shopping list to be able to make for several meals of that same dish.

3. Begin this practice with easy recipes that contain a relatively small amount of ingredients (so as not to overwhelm yourself or cause yourself to spend an excessive amount of time preparing the meals). Once you get in the habit, try more elaborate dishes.

4. If necessary, purchase quality freezer-, oven-, and microwave-safe containers of differing sizes, plus freezer tape. See Appendix C.

5. Consider investing in a three-in-one cooking system. See Appendix C.

TIP #38

Avoid multitasking while eating. That means no eating in front of the TV, or while talking on the phone.

These days, people are so busy that most continually attempt to do more than one activity at a time. Multitasking while we eat is particularly problematic. We check emails while consuming breakfast, continue to work while scarfing down a sandwich at lunch and relax by eating dinner or snacking in front of the TV.

Aside from diminishing our enjoyment of meals and depriving our brains and bodies of the breaks we periodically need, distracted eating can also lead to weight gain. Without purposely paying attention to our foods when dining, we can easily fall into the pattern of overeating. Slowing down, observing, savoring, and appreciating food can perpetuate better control of our intake.

Research confirms this theory. A 2013 report published in the American Journal of Clinical Nutrition provides a review of the research on eating style and its effect on attention and memory. Those scientists learned two valuable lessons: #1: Distraction during meals leads to consumption of more calories than when we give thought to what we're eating. #2: Paying attention to the foods we eat results in a reduction of intake after meals. In other words, subjects snacked less in the hours following a mindful vs a preoccupied dining experience.

When we're not concentrating our attention, it's easy to miss internal signals that inform us that we've eaten enough. It takes approximately 20 minutes for the brain to deliver the message that we have ingested enough food. While multitasking during meals, we tend to eat faster and finish eating all of the food in front of us, even if it's more than we need. And when we're not mindful of what we're consuming, apparently the fact that we have eaten already isn't stored in our memory banks, as noted by the researchers in the study mentioned above. As a result, we might eat again sooner, despite the fact that we aren't physically hungry.

Much discussion and written content indicate that mindful eating is the best way to lose weight and sustain a target weight (or range). Awareness of what we eat is important *when we're eating it*. But it goes beyond that.

Mindful eating means sensing the textures, aromas, flavors, and even the visual appeal of foods. Mindful practice intensifies our enjoyment of the food, and so we do not need as much to satisfy us.

Another interesting study focused solely on dessert. The findings suggested that we appreciate only the first two and then the last few bites of a given dessert. That makes a lot of sense, doesn't it? Imagine socializing with friends or family at dinner when the final course is placed in front of you. You will breathe in the aroma, look at this treat, and then reach for your fork. With that first bite, you think (or say), "Yum. This is tasty." After (or during) the second swallow, it's "Oh my gosh! This is scrumptious." The next thing you know, you're back to chatting and laughing with those friends or family members. Before you realize it, there's only one piece of that indulgence left on your plate. What do you do? You turn your awareness back to the dessert, savor the last bit, and think, "Boy, that was delicious!" Did you enjoy all of the mouthfuls in between? Probably not. So if you direct your attention, making a conscious decision to focus on your food, you just might find that, ultimately, a couple of bites will satisfy you. Mindful eating will allow you to recognize how unnecessary it is to eat every last morsel that is on your plate or in your bowl.

This newest challenge introduces one of the many ways to practice mindfulness. In this case, "mindful eating" will yield multiple benefits, one of which is weight reduction. Nevertheless, if multitasking while eating is your norm rather than the exception, I can understand that asking this of you may be a tall order. That being said, I'll remind you of one of my many mantras, hoping it inspires you to shift your habits, "Small changes, one at a time, lead to huge results!"

FOOD FOR THOUGHT... QUESTIONS & REFLECTIONS

1. List the activities that you typically pair with eating.

   _____
   _____
   _____
   _____
   _____
   _____
   _____

2. Imagine yourself eating but foregoing one or all of the activities you listed above. Reflect on the thoughts and emotions that arise as you envision that scenario.

   _____
   _____
   _____
   _____

3. How often do you pay attention to the aroma, texture, and taste of your food? What strategies might help remind you to do so more often?

4. On a scale of 1–10 (1=not at all, 10=I am ready and committed), how committed do you feel toward practicing mindfulness and not multitasking while eating?

5. What is the one small step you're willing to take in order to gradually cultivate the habit of mindful eating?

_____

_____

ACTION STEPS & EXERCISES

1. Every day of this week, commit to practicing mindful eating during one meal or snack time. Decide that you will not multitask, set aside the designated time to break away from other activities, and savor your food.

2. Only eat at a dining table during that one meal or snack, instead of at your desk, on the couch, in the car, etc.

3. Appreciate the appearance and fragrance of the food in front of you. Take one bite at a time; chew slowly. Put your fork down in between bites and pay attention to the taste and the sensations you feel while you eat.

4. Repeat this practice each day for your chosen meal or snack, and at the end of the week, take note of how you feel. You might like to journal about the experience.

5. Gradually add these practices and reflections to one more meal or snack at a time until mindful eating becomes routine.

TIP #39

When socializing, focus on the people, not the food.

I've coached many individuals who confided that there were times they skipped a party or social event because they didn't want to be tempted by indulgent foods they knew would be accessible. I completely understand their thought processes—most social gatherings include an abundance of goodies we would never bring into our homes, especially while trying to lose weight. And if we've successfully taken off pounds, there is the worry that we'll slip and regain. It's challenging to resist tempting foods when they're placed right in front of us, which is so often the case when we socialize outside of our own homes.

In spite of that, denying ourselves the enjoyable aspects of social gatherings isn't a useful strategy for permanent weight loss. If anything, missing out on the fun might very well make us feel resentful, sad, or deprived. And as a consequence, those emotions can send us right into our kitchens looking for comfort foods.

Why not shift focus, change our mindsets, and discover ways to enjoy social occasions without excessive worry about overeating? It is as simple as reminding ourselves that the purpose of these events is to reconnect with friends and family and appreciate our relationships, rather than fixating on the food.

When you find yourself in these situations, the following suggestions can help you avert the potential problem of overeating:

First and foremost, make sure you don't show up to a gathering famished. Typical behavior, but not productive, is assuming that you'll "save up" your calories for the party or event—meaning you'll forego lunch or eat very light meals or snacks throughout the day—and rationalize that such behavior will "balance out" your total caloric intake. This plan backfires when you walk into the get-together nearly ravenous, see all of the temptations, and end up consuming far more calories than you "saved up" during the day.

You think, "Well, I barely ate all day, so I don't have to worry about what I eat now." Often at social events, however, the choices of fare are higher in calories, sugar, and fat than the foods you usually consume. Where does that leave you? By then, you're so hungry that it becomes difficult to impossible to curb your appetite. Now you can see how essential it is to eat regular meals during the day and even have a healthy snack before leaving for the event. By doing so, you'll feel much more in control and make wiser choices.

Having done that, once you arrive at the affair, you can spend your time greeting other guests, getting involved in lively conversations, socializing, and simply enjoying the company of your friends and family. With your focus on the people rather than the food, you may even meet someone new and interesting.

Just as I expanded upon in Tip #14 (managing temptation when faced with a buffet), try to avoid standing or sitting near a display of food. Although that's where the majority of guests gather, you can suggest to whomever you are with that moving to a different spot will allow you to hear each other better. Now, if you still find yourself situated near food, for example, where bowls of nuts and chips abound, then it's a prime opportunity to tap into your mindfulness skills. Tell yourself, "Just because that food is there, it doesn't mean I need to eat it." (This might even serve as a jingle-like mantra you can whisper to yourself repeatedly if necessary.)

When it is time to eat, or you're truly feeling hungry, take a quick perusal of the available fare. Choose the foods you will eat based on what you love or what you know are your host's specialties. No rule states you must sample every single dish offered. Research shows that the wider the variety of food, the greater the number of calories we consume. Employing awareness (of yourself, your environment, and your current circumstances) will make for better self-control. (Remember Tip #38 that tipped you off about some of the many advantages of mindful eating?)

Next, if possible, sit down to eat. Shift your attention to the food on your plate. Taste, appreciate, and savor. Put your fork down in between bites. Take a short break from eating, look at your companion rather than the food, and try not to converse while you eat. Slow down, eat a bit, then talk a bit. This way, you genuinely take pleasure in the socialization and the cuisine. By slowing down, you'll also notice when you've had enough. With a buffet style meal, excuse yourself and discard your plate and utensils, signaling to your brain that the meal is over. If seated at a dining table, slightly push your plate away from you, and put your napkin on top of it; an indication to both yourself and your host that you are sated.

I would be remiss if I didn't mention the concern many have regarding the flow of alcohol that usually happens at social gatherings. Some people decide to forgo the event altogether because of worry about the excessive calories from alcoholic drinks or the discomfort of not partaking. Rather than taking that approach, strategize in advance on how you will handle drinking (or not).

There are two drawbacks to drinking alcoholic beverages when attempting weight loss. For starters, many mixed drinks include high-sugar, calorie-laden juices or syrups. Even if you choose wine, beer, or a shot worth of liquor with club soda, you very well may end up drinking excessive calories above your food calories. Also, alcohol tends to lower our inhibitions, leading to motivation and focus on weight loss slipping.

So planning how you'll manage this dilemma is important. If you opt not to drink at all, stick to your guns and don't apologize if asked why you're not imbibing. Just state you prefer not to drink alcohol at this time. Or if that's too uncomfortable for you, carry a glass of club soda with a lime or lemon. No one will know the difference.

If you do decide you would like to partake in a few drinks, stick to lower-calorie options, as mentioned above, and balance those extra calories with your food intake. For example, if you want a few drinks, decide you'll skip bread or dessert (or both). Try a full glass of water or seltzer in between each alcoholic drink. That's a great strategy for staying hydrated (since liquor is dehydrating), keeping you feeling satiated, and slowing down to decrease the number of drinks you have.

A lesson to be learned from Tip #39 (and quite a few of the other tips in this guidebook) is that the process of losing weight doesn't have to bring about feelings of deprivation. You're not "on a diet"; you're simply changing your habits. And the more you practice, the easier it gets. So the next time invited to a social event, agree to attend and put this tip into play. "Play" at the party and continue the celebration when you lose a few pounds!

FOOD FOR THOUGHT... QUESTIONS & REFLECTIONS

1. In the past, what have been your thoughts and behaviors concerning food temptations at social gatherings?

   _____

   _____

   _____

   _____

   _____

2. Have you ever forgone an event for fear of giving in to eating excessive calories? How did you feel about that?

   _____

   _____

   _____

   _____

3. What ideas do you have or strategies might you adopt to handle food temptations at social gatherings?

_____

_____

_____

_____

_____

_____

_____

_____

ACTION STEPS & EXERCISES

1. Take a look at your calendar and note any upcoming social engagements you may have. If they're ones you believe you would enjoy, commit to attending.

2. Anticipate in advance any challenges concerning food that you may encounter. (Examples: Will it be buffet style service? Will your best friend's famous apple pie be offered?) Come up with strategies in advance that will help you remain in control of your intake.

3. Abandon the notion (and practice) of "saving up calories" before special events. Eat light and healthy fare throughout the day leading up to occasions. Instead of skipping the parties and gatherings, skip the counterproductive habit of showing up hungry.

TIP #40

Paint your kitchen and dining room, and buy plates and utensils in soft hues such as blue, green, or gray.

Did you know that the color of one's dining area and even the color of plates and utensils can affect one's appetite? Studies indicate that while bright colors stimulate the appetite, surrounding ourselves with soft hues will do the opposite and suppress hunger.

When attempting to lose weight, though, we're so focused on what we should and should not eat that we pay little to no attention to additional elements at play. An important, yet often overlooked body of research tells us it's easier to change our eating environments than it is to alter our eating behaviors.

The colors around us make a considerable difference in some of our behaviors because they evoke our emotions. Countless studies have proven that colors significantly influence our minds and, hence, our actions. We can use this knowledge to our advantage when it comes to weight reduction.

The extent to which pigments and shades are linked with an individual's appetite is amazing. Some hues sway a person towards eating while others cause them to feel less hungry. Soft colors, for example blue, gray, and green, as well as dark tones, like brown and black, seem to diminish appetite.

For instance, of all the colors in the spectrum, blue has been proven to be unappetizing. Blue, it seems, acts as an appetite suppressant. Interestingly, we rarely see natural foods in the color blue. There are no blue leafy vegetables (blue lettuce?), no blue meats, and, aside from blueberries and a few varieties of blue-purple potatoes, blue pigments just do not exist in any significant quantities when it comes to food. Similarly, gray and brown don't often figure into edibles produced by Mother Nature.

Soft colors also tend to impact our moods; they calm and relax us. Those emotions are not shown to induce a strong desire to eat. And that's one of the reasons you rarely see a restaurant decorated in those tints.

On the other end of the spectrum (no pun intended!),

bright colors such as red, turquoise, yellow, and green stimulate appetite and have been proven to cue us to think about food. Essentially, they increase hunger. These particular colors create feelings of happiness and vitality, emotions associated with socializing and eating. Envision McDonalds' giant golden arches practically inviting (luring?) us to come in for a "happy" meal.

Red increases hunger by boosting metabolism, which is why red is such a popular color in restaurants. Think about the use of red in the logos and decor of popular fast food chains such as Dairy Queen, KFC, Burger King, and Pizza Hut just to name a few. What about the traditional red and white design of the Italian Trattorias found throughout the country, if not the world? Those decorating decisions were not made randomly; they were researched and implemented accordingly.

Those same bright colors can be seen in the food products we purchase at the grocery store. Manufacturers often use them to package foods for good reason (well, good reason on their parts—if color can influence our buying habits, you can be sure that producers will use it to their advantage).

Why not leverage this information to help you avoid overeating or eating for purposes other than physical hunger—the body's signal that it needs fuel? Of course, you can't control the colors in the restaurants you frequent, or the packaging of foods you like to purchase. Nonetheless, a simple *awareness* that colors affect people will result in more mindfulness in the decisions you do make.

The choice you *do have the ability to control* is the environment in which you eat in your home. **Consider painting your kitchen or dining room a soft, calming color.** Purchase plates and serving platters in blue, gray, or brown tones. If you can make subtle changes in your surroundings that impact how much or how little you eat, you'll see for yourself how bright the benefits can be!

FOOD FOR THOUGHT...
QUESTIONS & REFLECTIONS

1. Have you ever given thought to how color might impact your appetite and food choices? How might the information from this tip heighten your awareness of your surroundings when you are making food decisions?

   _____

   _____

   _____

   _____

   _____

2. Which is the liveliest, most enjoyable restaurant you like to frequent? Do you believe color and decor effect your mood and food choices when you're there?

   _____

   _____

   _____

   _____

3. What are your favorite colors? How do those colors make you feel emotionally?

_____

_____

_____

_____

ACTION STEPS & EXERCISES

1. For the next week, take note of the color and decor of all the places where you eat—your home, your office lunch room, the restaurants you frequent, etc.

2. If you decide that changing the colors in your home eating areas is a wise decision, create a comfortable budget to work within. Plan the modifications you will make and when you can make them. (Repaint the kitchen, buy new plates and utensils, change the rug in the dining room, purchase new tablecloths, etc.)

3. Begin to take note of the colors around you when visiting friends' and relatives' homes or restaurants. Use your new awareness to help you make wise decisions concerning your food choices and satiating your appetite.

TIP #41

Designate the kitchen as a room to be used only for food prep and eating.

One sure method to reduce the number of calories we consume each day is cutting back on mindless eating. That is, when we reach for food, not because we're physically hungry, but because our environments (or something within them) trigger the urge to eat. In my opinion, a tremendous amount of mindless eating occurs in the kitchen, where we often spend time busy with activities other than preparing or consuming a meal or snack.

When we're distracted or multitasking, we fail to put much thought into our actions; we reach for food and proceed to ingest it. Sometimes we eat without paying any attention whatsoever, never even realizing that we are biting, chewing, or swallowing. Have you ever been reading the newspaper or talking on the phone and, when finished, you "discover" that you just polished off a bag of chips? (Yes, the one your kids left on the kitchen counter.)

If we spend lots of time in our kitchens engaged in other activities that have nothing to do with food preparation or eating, there's a good chance that we will end up consuming excess calories.

In his book, *Slim by Design: Mindless Eating Solutions for Everyday Life*, doctor and author Brian Wansink addresses just this topic. He states, "The more you hang out in your kitchen, the more you'll eat." As a leading researcher in eating behavior, a professor at Cornell University, and the Director of Cornell's Food and Brand Lab, Dr. Wansink is truly an expert on what factors influence our eating habits.

Every aspect of the kitchen reminds us of food: the smells, the appliances, the cabinets, and the items on our counters—both foodstuffs and that which we use to prepare food. And, of course, the kitchen is the room we associate with meals. It's the place we go when we need or want a snack or drink.

Why is it, then, that so many of us gravitate toward the kitchen for non-meal-related tasks? Why do we remain in the same room after a meal for much more time than we should?

In many homes, the kitchen is the sunniest, most spacious area. Since we associate that space with family meals or friends gathering around the table, it feels warm, welcoming, and comforting all-around.

Friends pop in for a quick hello, and we lead them straight to the kitchen. We encourage our children to do homework in the kitchen so that we're accessible in case they need help—perhaps while we prepare a meal or attend to our own work. We sort our mail at the dining table. Time for a family meeting? We meet at the kitchen table.

In theory, therefore, the kitchen seems like an ideal room in which to "hang out." But if you're trying to lose weight or even just cut back on consuming unnecessary and often unhealthy calories, the kitchen is not a place where you want to spend the majority of your day. That being said, with all of the other areas in the house to choose from, why do we keep finding ourselves in that particular room?

Whether we realize it or not (and hopefully now you will), the layout of our homes encourages us to spend our time in the kitchen.

Almost all homes have a back door that leads directly into the kitchen. It's as if that one room is inviting us to spend more time there than anywhere else.

Modern architecture incorporates open kitchens that lead right into family rooms, where we usually find a TV. So while we watch, the kitchen is in plain sight and easily accessible. During our favorite programs, we're frequently bombarded with food commercials that trigger a desire to eat. Couple those cues with tempting treats a mere few steps away, and it is easy to understand why we munch despite a lack of actual hunger.

Many kitchens have a corner cabinet with a built-in desk: an ideal (or maybe not so ideal) place to keep a computer, the family calendar, tend to our bills and tackle our paperwork.

However, if weight loss is a priority, it's well worth it to heighten awareness of our environment and how it can encourage the consumption of excess calories. Since awareness is the first step towards change and now that you're enlightened, let's give this some thought.

Think about the times you find yourself in the kitchen involved in an activity that's in no way related to cooking or eating. Where else might you carry out that same activity? Is there a way you can take the good feelings you get from your kitchen into another room?

I did just that by creating a corner in my living room—an underused but beautiful space where I can read or chat on the phone. I purchased a comfortable and sleek recliner to face my big picture window, placed a small table nearby, and installed a phone jack as well. It's one of my favorite spots, my private escape. Perhaps you have ideas to create a special nook for yourself (and your family) other than in the kitchen.

As a work-from-home entrepreneur, I also have an area earmarked as an office where I keep my paperwork. In it, my desk faces the window. With plants on the desk and throughout the room, that space feels inviting as well.

As you read this tip, are you conjuring up any ideas to help "get out of the kitchen"? Are there some activities you routinely do there that might be delegated to another room in your home? Even a slight decrease of time spent in your kitchen may result in a big reduction in the total calories you ingest each day.

Perhaps you already have a desk in your kitchen, and it's the only place you can feasibly work. Then the job of modifying your behavior becomes slightly more challenging. Don't despair. Simply be aware that remaining in the kitchen can result in mindless eating. Establish a rule that no food will be allowed on or near your desk, and that you'll only "allow" yourself to eat at the dining table (remember, no standing). If you find yourself thinking about food, stop and ask, "Am I really hungry?" If the answer is no, get back to work. If that fails, take a break. Leave the kitchen and tackle another task elsewhere. Wait until the urge to eat subsides before returning to your work in the kitchen.

The more you train yourself to identify the sensations of actual physical hunger, the easier it will be for you to resist cues that are coming from the environment, not your physiology. The more you heighten your awareness of how the environment can hinder or support your weight loss journey, the better you'll get at setting yourself up for success.

What does Tip #41—and for that matter, all 52 Tips—boil down to? The more you shift your behaviors, the closer you'll come to *mastering the inner game of weight loss* without going on a diet.

I encourage you to learn more about how you can alter your environment to control your appetite by reading the fascinating research that Dr. Wansink shares in his book, *Slim by Design: Mindless Eating Solutions for Everyday Life*. To view a sample and order a copy, see Appendix A.

In Tip #42, we'll continue to explore additional ways you can support your efforts by shaping your surroundings.

FOOD FOR THOUGHT... QUESTIONS & REFLECTIONS

1. How often do you think you engage in mindless eating while "hanging out in the kitchen"?

   _____

   _____

2. In what way does it influence your daily caloric intake?

   _____

   _____

3. Do you believe reducing the amount of time you spend in the kitchen would impact your weight loss goals? Why or why not?

   _____

   _____

   _____

   _____

ACTION STEPS & EXERCISES

1. Write down all the activities you typically engage in while in the kitchen that aren't related to meal preparation or consumption of meals and snacks.

   _____

   _____

   _____

   _____

   _____

   _____

2. How might you reshape your environment to support your efforts to cut back on the amount of time you spend in your kitchen, engaged in activities unrelated to food preparation and consumption?

   _____

   _____

   _____

   _____

3. Write down the one action step you're ready and committed to take in order to reduce the amount of time you currently spend in your kitchen during the course of a typical day.

_____

_____

_____

TIP #42

Replace oversized plates, bowls, and glasses with smaller ones.

Throughout the past several chapters, I've described how and why the environment can impact not only your food choices, but also the extent to which you eat (regarding volume, calories and nutrient-rich—or non-nutritious—fare). I've shared scientific evidence, examples from my own experience (personally and as a wellness coach), and overall suggestions based on same to help illustrate, guide, and motivate you toward adapting your environment to foster, as opposed to sabotaging, your weight loss efforts.

In that same vein, in Tip #42, I will continue this dialogue by highlighting the benefits of replacing oversized dining ware with smaller pieces. If you could reduce the number of calories you consume and still feel satisfied at the end of a meal, would you take advantage of that excellent opportunity? That's what this strategy can do for you, and it's easy!

Logic dictates that, if you use a larger-sized plate, you will put more food on it. It's as if the plate is "giving you permission" to consume more—servings seem skimpy when there's too much space left on the plate, right? When you consider putting a cup of mashed potatoes onto a 12-inch or 10-inch plate, it will appear as if there's much less food on it than when spooning the same amount onto an 8-inch plate.

And if you put more food on your plate or in your bowl, or you drink from larger glasses and mugs, there's an awfully good chance you will be consuming more calories. We tend to eat with our eyes, not our stomachs; more often than not, we clean our plates even when our stomachs have had enough.

Research supports this rationale and presents a relatively solid case for substituting oversized tableware with moderately-sized pieces.

A review of 58 studies provides fascinating information on precisely this topic. In those many studies, researchers captured data from over 6,600 subjects. What they yielded was convincing evidence that people consume more food when offered larger portions *or* when they eat from bigger plates, bowls, glasses, and cups. In fact, the scientists from the University of Cambridge predicted that if we consistently reduced our exposure to larger-sized portions, packaging, or tableware, the average daily energy consumed (in other terms, calories) from food can decrease by 22–29 percent among adults in the US and 12–16 percent among adults in the UK.

Dr. Brian Wansink, author of *Slim by Design: Mindless Eating Solutions for Everyday Life*, tested this same principle, using smaller plates in his research laboratory. Not only did he find that his participants cut their caloric intake, but they also expressed that they felt equally as full as those subjects who ate from the larger plates. In essence, you trick your brain into feeling just as satisfied with less food.

Where am I taking you here? I propose you begin by consciously making changes in your environment to make it work for you. It's way easier than always trying to depend on willpower to control your intake. Give serious consideration to trading in your oversized plates, bowls, and glasses for smaller ones. If you typically eat cereal, soup, or ice cream from larger than standard-sized bowls, research now proves that you likely eat oversized portions of those same—and similar—foods. Same holds true for liquid calories—those from juice, milk, smoothies, etc. We consume more when using short, wide glasses than skinny ones. So, not only are you ingesting more calories than you need to fuel yourself adequately, but you're also taking in more than the amount of food you need to feel sated.

For so many of my clients, and probably for you too, weight gain slowly crept up over the years. Thus, the weight loss struggle began. Much of the reason for this is due to the changes that have taken place in lifestyle, society, and environments. We're constantly bombarded with subtle (or sometimes not-so-subtle) cues to eat, and eat, and eat. One of the detriments of technology is that it has promoted less physical activity than in the generations before us. Marketers send us the message that more and bigger is always better.

But as Dr. Wansink says in his book, "The good news is that the same levers that almost invisibly lead you to slowly gain weight can be pushed in the other direction to just as invisibly lead you to slowly lose weight. If we don't realize we're eating a little less than we need, we don't feel deprived. If we don't feel deprived, we're less likely to backslide and find ourselves overeating to compensate for everything we've forgone."

I believe that the doctor's statement sums up much of what I have conveyed. As such—and with some of the real evidence I offer in Tip #42, not to mention within many chapters of Mastering the Inner Game of Weight Loss—utilizing these tools incrementally will take you a long way along your path to weight loss. And that is some oversized news to help you on your way to "undersizing" your weight!

FOOD FOR THOUGHT... QUESTIONS & REFLECTIONS

1. Think about the dining ware you use in your home and other locations where you typically eat. Would you consider those dishes to be standard or oversized?

   _____

   _____

   _____

   _____

   _____

2. In what way has the size of plates and bowls impacted your portion control?

   _____

   _____

   _____

   _____

   _____

3. What are some approaches you can take to assure portion control when dining at home and in other environments?

_____

_____

_____

_____

_____

ACTION STEPS & EXERCISES

1. If you're unsure of the sizes of your plates and bowls (in diameter), go ahead and measure them.

2. If you discover they're larger-sized tableware such as mentioned above, experiment for one week with using smaller plates, bowls, and glasses. Utilize inexpensive paper or plastic, rather than rushing out to purchase new. Journal about the experience, paying close attention to how satisfied you feel (or not) at the conclusion of a meal or snack.

3. **OPTIONAL:** Weigh yourself at the beginning of the trial week before you begin using smaller tableware. Weigh yourself after seven days of forgoing oversized plates. Have the results been positive?

4. If you feel ready to commit to replacing your dining ware with a smaller set, schedule a date to go shopping! (You certainly don't need to seek out extremely miniature-sized tableware, if it even exists! Nor do you need to bust your budget!)

5. Check out the resources in Appendix C for purchasing tableware that has portion control built in. There are many fun, good looking, and inexpensive options available.

TIP #43

Keep healthy foods in clear containers and bowls, on counters and at eye level in the fridge.

Do you remember the chapter in which I referenced the adage, "Out of sight, out of mind"? I set out to substantiate how and why that saying holds true with respect to eating behavior. Essentially, when we see tempting treats, we're more inclined to eat them. So let's dig in (wink, wink) to this notion a bit further.

There are so many delicious and nutritious foods we can enjoy every day; choices that will keep us fueled properly, feeling satisfied, and contribute to good health and weight loss. The trick is to have them accessible and—best case scenario—visible!

Often, we reach for nutrient-poor junk foods simply because they are easily available and, frequently right in front of us. Whether it's time for a snack or meal, when we are ready to eat, it's way easier to make wise choices if the unhealthy fare is not staring us in the face.

When we're hungry, our instinct is to reach for food that is quick and easy. Unless there's a healthy alternative prepared and waiting in front of us, we will grab hold of just about any edible within sight. Most people will open the cabinets and seize the bag of chips, a couple of cookies, or a snack bar (which more often than not is merely a candy bar dressed up as health food). Typically hidden in our refrigerator drawers are the wiser choices, such as fruit, vegetables, or high-quality protein. Rarely are the wholesome foods sitting on our counters, visible and obtainable.

I am sure you can surmise, therefore, why I recommend that you buy lots more of the "good" rather than "bad" edibles. However, a common complaint from many clients is that, when they purchase produce, or deli meats such as sliced turkey or chicken breast, too often it goes bad before they have the chance to eat it. They find themselves discarding rotten fruits and vegetables and spoiled meats, aggravated because they wasted money. When I inquire about where those foods are kept, the prevailing answer is that they are stored "out of sight." Here, then, you have another benefit of keeping nutritious fare—especially perishables—noticeable: You'll waste less food and money. If you're worried that the visible temptation will lure you into eating too many fruits and vegetables and, thereby, increase your weight, let me reassure you that I've never met an individual who has grappled with extra pounds due to excess produce intake.

So set yourself up for success! Create an environment in which you're motivated to eat well. Remember, "Out of sight, out of mind. In sight, top of mind."

Here are some ideas to keep wholesome foods visible:

Lots of yummy fruits and veggies don't need to be refrigerated; they can sit on the counter or kitchen table in bowls. Keep apples, pears, bananas, and oranges in plain sight, so you will undoubtedly notice them. You can do the same with cherry tomatoes, baby carrots, and sugar snap peas as well. I do advise, however, that you place those bowls back in the fridge at the end of the day to extend the shelf-life of these gifts from Mother Nature.

For foodstuffs that must be kept cold, position a clear bowl of berries or cubed melon on the center shelf of your fridge, near your yogurt, cheese sticks, and cottage cheese. Store sliced turkey or chicken breasts in transparent containers as well. A few pieces of lean cold cuts make a satisfying, quick snack. Have your favorite nuts and seeds visible as well, but do be cautious about portion control. Despite being wonderfully nutritious snacks, nuts and seeds are high in calories, and it's very easy to over-consume if you take a handful each time you see them. I choose to buy pre-portioned, individually-sized packages of the nuts I enjoy. If you prefer not to splurge (they are a bit more expensive when sold that way), you can purchase large packages and portion them out into snack-sized baggies; it's probably best to get them into those baggies immediately after bringing them home. In other words, don't leave yourself open, tempted to eat larger portions.

Go ahead and bring those types of snacks to your workplace. Keep the items that do not need refrigeration out in the open on your desk. Store the rest in the office refrigerator if you're lucky enough to have one, or consider purchasing an inexpensive mini fridge or cooler for all for those nutritious treats. Snapping up such wholesome selections when you're hungry, because these foods are now so conspicuous and accessible, will raise your consumption of healthy fare and reduce the amount of time you rummage for higher calorie, less nutrient-rich edibles.

This tip also proves a great strategy if you're looking to encourage healthy eating choices in your household (or even your workplace). It's relatively common knowledge that we should consume a wide variety of fruits and vegetables every day, but unfortunately, most people don't come close to eating the recommended 5–11 servings of fruits and veggies daily. By taking advantage of Tip #43 at home, you'll increase your chances of meeting those guidelines, and it will have a ripple effect on those with whom you share your household. For instance, my husband would never think to eat fruit when he wants a snack. Inevitably, though, he'll eat some while walking by, if cut up apples, orange segments, or melon pieces are on the counter. I always keep a pint of rinsed cherry tomatoes, grapes, and strawberries in view. They're my daughter's first choices if she needs a nibble to curb hunger in between meals.

Is the takeaway pretty obvious—like the healthy food should be? All it takes is moving the non-nutritious junk food to the back of your cabinets and fridge, out of ready sight. And transfer the more nutritious fare to locations in your house and place of work where they're easily seen. Incorporate this simple approach into your routine and before long, you'll be fueling your body with high-quality, delicious, and nutritious foods; and your desire for junk food will diminish. You'll be a master of the game of weight loss, without having gone on a diet!

FOOD FOR THOUGHT...
QUESTIONS & REFLECTIONS

1. Where do you usually store your fruit? Your veggies? Your nuts and seeds?

   _____

   _____

   _____

   _____

2. Whether in or out of the fridge, in what kinds of platters, bowls, or containers do you keep those kinds of nutritious (and tasty) foods?

   _____

   _____

   _____

   _____

   _____

3. Which foodstuffs are you willing to experiment with by moving them to a more visible location?

_____
_____
_____
_____
_____
_____
_____

ACTION STEPS & EXERCISES

1. Set time aside to rearrange the foods in your cabinets and refrigerator. Put healthy food in clear, see-through containers or open dishes and bowls. Move the less nutritious fare to a place where it's not so easily spotted.

2. On your next trip to the market, fill your cart with a wide variety of fruits, vegetables, nuts, and seeds.

3. Once home, immediately upon unpacking your groceries, transfer those items to transparent containers and bowls, and place them at eye level in the fridge and on your counters.

4. Take mental note of—or write down—whether or not you find yourself eating more nutritiously after you've implemented this approach.

_____

_____

_____

_____

_____

_____

_____

TIP #44

Keep treats and temptations in opaque containers situated in the back of the refridgerator, freezer, or cabinets.

In an ideal world, we would keep all tempting, non-nutritious treats out of our homes and workplaces, especially while endeavoring to lose weight. Reality sneaks in, though, and makes it crystal clear that most of us live and work with other people who want those yummies available. And the truth is that we should be able to enjoy the occasional goodie despite the fact that we're attempting to slim down.

If you've been reading these guidebook chapters (aka, Tips) in sequence, you may have noticed that certain ones can precipitate offshoots, so to speak, which lead to even more weight loss strategies. Tip #44 is one of them. In it, I will stoke the conversation about the environment's impact on eating habits by adding another log to the fire.

Throughout this guidebook, I have not, and surely will not, suggest that you must rid your house of all treats when you're trying to lose weight. That is impractical on several levels. After all, your family members may resent the absence of cookies, chips, and ice cream. In addition, you might like to reserve a few edible extravagances for hosting guests. And, as suggested above, you yourself might make the conscious decision to enjoy an occasional indulgence, which, by the way, is A-OK. "Stashing" some "guilty pleasures" in your house can still be part of a healthy weight loss regimen—"stashing," perhaps, being the operative word. As long as you remain aware of your actions (eating mindfully), and adjust your environment to minimize temptation, an occasional treat fits into a well-rounded, healthy dietary plan.

Nonetheless, if you have high-caloric foods staring you in the face every time you walk into your kitchen or family room—whether on a counter or table, or even when you open the fridge or freezer—it becomes much more difficult to say "no."

So here we examine the essence of Tip #43—keeping highly nutritious foods, such as fruits, veggies, and high-quality protein within sight and reach—from a somewhat different angle. We've already determined that whether or not you see particular foods first plays a significant role in whether or not you will eat them. It follows, therefore, that when high-calorie, non-nutritious yummies remain less visible, you'll elect to eat them less often. This is when the adage "out of sight, out of mind" applies.

How can you slightly maneuver your surroundings so that resisting temptations becomes easier? First, if you don't already have them, purchase opaque containers and a roll of freezer tape. That way, you can effectively "hide" those sweet tidbits and highly caloric indulgences, and label the containers so you and your family can still identify them later. Second, place the containers in the back of your cabinets and deep in your refrigerator and freezer drawers. Follow suit for leftover pastries, such as cake, cupcakes, and home baked cookies; that fare freezes beautifully. Set them in the far reaches of the freezer, labeled with the containers' contents. Third, make sure that the frozen veggies, poultry, and lean meats are the first foods you see when you open the fridge and freezer.

If dishes or bowls sitting on your counters, tables, or desk are filled with candy or another tempting foodstuff, pack them away and replace them with decorative items or healthy snacks such as fruits or veggies. When you make the deliberate decision to "allow yourself" a treat (which, again, is perfectly fine), you'll have to work just a bit harder to access it or similar kinds of goodies. You'll need to dig deep into the rear sections of the refrigerator, freezer, drawers, or pantry to retrieve what you want. Then you can apportion an appropriate serving, enjoy it, savor it, and finally replace that container back in its spot. "Out of sight, out of mind."

This approach may not completely prevent you from reaching for the foods that don't promote weight loss, but I assure you it will reduce your intake. And as is inherent in my mantra (or one of many mantras), making shifts in small increments will yield significant benefits. When you arrange your home so that tasty, nutritious foods are in plain sight and empty-calorie foods are left out of sight, you'll be much more inclined to choose foods that lead you closer and closer to attaining your goals. Add this tip to your weight loss toolbox and, little by little, you'll advance yourself along the road toward *mastering the inner game of weight loss without going on a diet*.

FOOD FOR THOUGHT... QUESTIONS & REFLECTIONS

1. What types of high-calorie "treats" do you typically keep in your home? Where and in what kinds of containers do you store them?

   _____

   _____

   _____

   _____

   _____

   _____

2. In what environments other than your home do you find yourself faced with weight-loss-sabotaging foodstuffs? (e.g., office kitchen, hair salon, social gatherings, etc.) How do you commonly respond to those temptations?

   _____

   _____

   _____

3. How might you set up your environment so that you are "faced" with the decision to indulge or bypass foods that do not support your weight loss efforts less often?

ACTION STEPS & EXERCISES

1. Take stock of the foods you currently have in your home that don't help you stay the course on your weight loss journey. Reorganize them in opaque containers, in locations where they aren't easy to see and/or access.

2. If you don't currently have opaque storage containers or freezer tape, set out to purchase them.

3. If you haven't already done so, place healthy foods where they are visible (see Tip #43).

4. Take mental note—or better yet, write down—whether or not you see a shift in the types of foods and frequency you reach for them after you've made these simple adjustments.

_____

_____

_____

_____

_____

_____

_____

TIP #45

Use positive self-talk, mantras, and visual reminders of your goals.

Tip #45 is one you may find quite challenging, although, in truth, it is easy to slip into your everyday life. Some individuals, however, feel it uncomfortable and difficult to implement (at least in the beginning). Why? Because when it comes to weight loss, or maintaining weight loss, most people have been repeating particular stories for years—often in the form of negative internal self-talk. Changing that story to an empowering one rather than a sabotaging one can be quite difficult. Old habits die hard.

Does any of this mind chatter sound familiar?

"I don't have the willpower to resist fattening foods."
"I'll probably fail this time, just like I have every other."
"This is just too hard."
"I have a slow metabolism. Everyone in my family has the fat gene."
"It's useless."
"I blew it."
"I'm such a loser."

I've rarely had a client who didn't express some version of these narratives over and over again (out loud or to themselves). Unfortunately, the tales we tell ourselves are usually what unfolds in real life. This notion is reminiscent of the wise observation coined by Henry Ford, "Whether you think you can or you think you can't, you are right."

What's the takeaway with regard to weight loss? Well, changing the storylines in your head and talking back to that negative mind chatter (which, by the way, represents your own voice) plays a significant role in whether one succeeds at losing weight. Yes, you DO have control over your self-talk, your thoughts, and the actions that follow.

A mantra is a word, sound, or phrase that one repeats to him- or herself while meditating; the mantra helps the meditator concentrate. Mantras and positive self-talk can be employed at any time to aid us in remaining focused on long-range goals. Stating them, out loud if possible, can feel awkward at first. In the case of Tip #45, then, if disputing negative narratives feels forced, you may just need to "fake it until you make it." With practice, saying positive statements and affirmations begin to feel natural and empowering.

Let me give some examples of self-sabotaging mind chatter transformed into positive statements or affirmations. If you hear yourself saying (or thinking), "Every time I've lost weight, I've never been able to keep it off." simply add to the chatter, "Up until now."

Or your inner voice might egg you on (no pun intended!): "Gosh I really want one of those cupcakes. Eating only one won't hurt." Reply to it with, "No, I am not hungry. I want to lose the excess pounds I've been carrying around, and I *can* resist temptation."

Many people are particularly fond of this affirmative statement: "Nothing tastes as good as having a strong lean body!" Along those lines, you can also try, "Only high-quality fuel goes into my healthy, efficient body." Or how about a mantra I happen to love? "Don't give up what you want the most for what you want right now."

There are countless mantras and affirmations you can use to inspire yourself. Play with them, create new ones, and stick with the ones that resonate: what suit and truly motivate you.

Visual cues can be extraordinarily helpful reminders of goals and aspirations as well. I use a very personal cue—one that's close to me in heart and mind. I have a very specific image that keeps me highly motivated to exercise daily. In my office, there is a photo of me riding a horse when I was in Colorado. It is a snapshot taken during one of my favorite vacations. It reminds me how much I want to stay powerful and healthy so that I can continue participating in the activities I so enjoy, such as horseback riding and hiking. Merely glancing at that picture encourages me to stand up, leave my office and head to the gym, even when I didn't feel the urge beforehand.

If you have a favorite picture of yourself, from a time when you felt thinner and more comfortable in your body, post it in a prominent location. It will reinforce the fact that you had been slimmer in the past and can become slimmer yet again. Or cut pictures from magazines that inspire you and remind you of why you want to lose weight. One of my clients placed a beautiful photo of her children on the kitchen shelf. Each time she looks at it, she pairs it with the mantra, "I am getting strong and healthy to be there for my children, and to be a role model for living a healthy lifestyle." It's no coincidence that this same client has since lost 50 pounds and sustained that weight for over a year, to date.

Again, for some people, Tip #45 presents a bit of a challenge. It feels awkward and uncomfortable to tell yourself a "story" you may not yet believe is true. At the same time, this strategy centers upon overcoming some of the impediments any of us might have while attempting to lose weight. As George S. Patton once said, **"Accept the challenges so that you can feel the exhilaration of victory."**

FOOD FOR THOUGHT... QUESTIONS & REFLECTIONS

1. What are some of the negative "stories" you tell yourself regarding your personality and abilities, particularly, but not necessarily concerning your body image and weight loss?

   _____

   _____

   _____

   _____

   _____

   _____

   _____

   _____

   _____

   _____

   _____

   _____

2. Read the statements you just wrote down out loud. What emotions and feelings arise when you talk to or about yourself in that manner?

_____

_____

_____

_____

_____

_____

_____

_____

_____

_____

_____

_____

_____

_____

3. Rewrite the above statements, changing them into positive, encouraging affirmations.

4. Look at framed pictures or those in photo albums you have in your house. Choose one or more of yourself when you were thinner, stronger, and healthier all-around. How do you feel when you see the image?

_____

_____

_____

_____

_____

_____

ACTION STEPS & EXERCISES

1. Create a mantra or positive affirmation that feels empowering and begin using it daily. Google motivational quotes for inspiration and ideas. Write it down below.

_____

_____

_____

2. This week, notice your mind chatter. If it's negative or sabotaging, experiment in "turning it around" so that it becomes positive and motivating. Speak your new statements out loud (better yet, in front of the mirror), in a whisper, or think them silently.

3. Write down your new favorite mantras and place them in areas where you'll see them frequently (e.g., on index cards to put in your wallet, stuck to your mirror, or on your office desk).

4. Choose your visual cues and put them into prominent places, as above.

TIP #46

Ask those you love and trust for the support and encouragement you need in order to succeed in your weight loss efforts.

Over the many past chapters, we've addressed an array of weight reduction strategies you can employ to help you help yourself. Note that most of those approaches encompass changes you can make to your environment and behaviors you can modify (which includes removing self-sabotaging habits). Please be very aware, however, that asking for aid and inspiration from close family, friends, and coworkers are of equal, if not higher, importance.

Quite often, those around us hamper our efforts without realizing they're doing so. Consider these hypothetical scenarios: Your spouse brings home your favorite ice cream flavor. Your mother encourages you to take a second helping because she "made it just for you." A colleague bakes brownies every Friday and offers you one, two, or even three of them. Friends persuade you to skip the gym and join them at a happy hour instead. The list goes on and on and on.

When I work with clients on the subject of communication, I frequently need to tell them, "No one is a mind reader." We can't assume that others know or understand what it is we need and want. The only way to make one's wishes known is to explain oneself. And what I mean is to be unambiguous in your explanation. Don't speak in "hint" language—be clear and concise about what you want and need to succeed with your weight loss efforts.

That being said, I understand and empathize with people who don't feel comfortable talking about their weight loss endeavors (even with their loved ones). If you happen to be an individual who fears judgment; being monitored and nagged; or becoming a disappointment if you don't succeed at what you've set out to accomplish, you may then choose to go it alone.

However, there are plenty of ways to enlist support without announcing to the world, "I'm going on a diet," or "I want to lose weight." Learning how to speak up in a way that is comfortable and gets you the support needed to be successful, is crucial. Otherwise, you'll find yourself often faced with situations like those mentioned, and so many more. The type of circumstances that can lead you to feel annoyed and resentful; emotions that don't make this journey easy to navigate!

If you've been reading this guidebook and have begun implementing the tips described in its pages, you've chosen to embark on a path that will effect a series of lifestyle changes. This time around, you're not going on yet another diet. So when discussing your new behaviors and choices with others, shift the focus from weight loss to your aspiration of living more healthily. Certainly, no one can argue with an individual who states "I've decided to start eating more nutritiously," "I want to cut back on sugar," or "my objective is to be in better shape."

Now that you can appreciate how it is to your benefit to open up communications, how can or should you begin? First, you need to gather your thoughts; precisely explain what it is you do and *don't* want from the people around you. Be clear. Be firm. And don't let frustration or anger get in the way.

Let's take a closer look at some of the examples above and expand on them to include effective—but not forceful—communication:

If you're married, convey to your spouse how much you appreciate his or her thoughtfulness, but that you're trying to cut back on calories and non-nutritious food. In an even and pleasing tone, ask him or her not to buy ice cream or any of your "trigger foods." Tell Mom how much you love the fact that she goes out of her way to cook your favorite dishes, but that you are full. Ask if she would wrap leftovers for you to take home and enjoy for lunch the next day. (Some people refer to it as a "care package," and it fits in light of this Tip, right?) Let your coworker know you're grateful for her generosity, but the sugary treats she brings in are so delicious that they're too hard to resist. Explain the "sugar rush" you get from eating them makes you hyperactive, and so it becomes difficult for you to focus on your work. Enthusiastically, suggest she leave the goodies in the staff kitchen where everyone can enjoy them. When it comes time to choose between the gym and happy hour, let your friends know how much of a priority it is that you fit in exercise and this is the only time of day you can go. If they try to cajole you, stand firm in your decision. Tell them you'll meet them afterward, or perhaps, invite them to join you at the gym!

You may find yourself angry or frustrated by "helpful" comments such as, "Are you sure you want to eat that?" Or, "Didn't you say you wanted to go to the gym today?" Gently but firmly let those "helpful" folks know that those sorts of questions are not so helpful. Even remarks, such as "You look like you lost weight. Good for you," might make you uncomfortable. Maybe you simply don't like having attention called to yourself. In those situations, again, you'll need to be open by sharing what kinds of questions and statements are—*and are not*—to your benefit.

Explain what you *do want*. Perhaps you *do want* your significant other to push you out of bed in the mornings so you can get in a workout rather than let you hit the snooze button. Maybe you'll find it more helpful if friends do take notice when you're sticking to your healthy eating plan, and you would appreciate them applauding your discipline and willpower. If you typically put your children to bed, request that your spouse takes over that responsibility so you can attend an exercise class.

On the path to weight loss and maintenance, it's more

than likely you'll find it difficult to stay the course if you try to go it alone. Enlist the help of family and friends you trust. Show them you love them by opening up communication, and they'll follow suit by doing the same. (As the saying goes, "It can't hurt to ask.")

FOOD FOR THOUGHT... QUESTIONS & REFLECTIONS

1. In the past, when you attempted to make healthy lifestyle changes, in what ways have you shared your objectives with friends, family, and coworkers?

   _____
   _____
   _____
   _____
   _____
   _____

2. On a scale of 1–10, (1= not at all comfortable, 10= totally comfortable) how comfortable are you discussing your weight loss efforts with others around you? If you rated a 5 or below, why do you think that is so? What would you need to do in order to increase your comfort level?

   _____
   _____

_____

_____

_____

_____

_____

3. Brainstorm a list of all the things you would like significant individuals in your life to do/say, and not do/say, in order to support and encourage your weight loss efforts.

_____

_____

_____

_____

_____

_____

_____

_____

_____

ACTION STEPS & EXERCISES

1. Write down the names of all the folks you're in contact with frequently, the people who matter to you most, and those who you see very often; and who can potentially help or hinder your efforts.

2. Make a list of what you would like them to do, and what you would prefer they not do, in order to support you on your journey.

_____

_____

_____

_____

_____

_____

_____

_____

_____

_____

_____

_____

_____

3. Next, schedule a time for a heart-to-heart talk, preferably where you won't be distracted or interrupted.

4. At that "meeting," in a clear and calm manner, describe what it is he or she can do to support you. In that same tone of voice, request the assistance and encouragement you would appreciate as you embark on your weight loss journey.

TIPS #47–#50

Mint, mint, mint, and more mint. Use mint to boost your weight reduction efforts: inhale, ingest, brush, and chew.

This chapter is unique from all of the rest in that I have combined Tips #47 through #50. Why? Because this series of tips encompass several approaches with one common denominator: all revolve around what can be a weight watcher's best friend, **MINT**. Yes, I'm referring to the aromatic herb mint, found in so many edible and inedible forms!

Two of the greatest challenges we encounter when we attempt to shed pounds is insatiable hunger and fighting the food cravings that often emerge as your body acclimates to existing on fewer calories. Voracious appetites and difficulty resisting cravings are, of course, detriments to weight loss. Did you know that something as simple to obtain as mint can come to your rescue? Not only that, but you can reap the benefits of this handy herb in more than one way!

Food and weight management experts are aware that some of Mother Nature's comestibles, including various herbs, serve as natural appetite suppressants; yet with none of the side effects or hazards of the "magic potions" some manufacturers market via retail or internet channels.

Studies indicate that, despite the fact that the positive effects it produces are primarily psychological, *mint works*. You can easily derive the payoffs mint provides by using it in different forms:

- **Tip #47:** Inhale the aroma of the mint leaves themselves. Lavish in lotions infused with its essence, or burn mint-scented candles in the kitchen and dining room. In other words, breathe in its powerful, pleasing fragrance to suppress your appetite.

- **Tip #48:** Ingest peppermint tea or water

flavored with mint, or pop a pre- or post-meal, sugar-free mint into your mouth to curtail cravings.

- **Tip #49:** Brush your teeth with mint-flavored toothpaste or use mint-flavored floss after you eat to control cravings and signal the end of a meal.

- **Tip #50:** Chew sugarless mint gum between meals to diminish both hunger and cravings.

Dr. Bryan Raudenbush, an Associate Professor of Psychology at Wheeling Jesuit University in West Virginia, discovered that inhaling the scent of peppermint can help you sidestep afternoon munchies. In his preliminary research, subjects who periodically sniffed mint throughout the day ate an average of 3,000 fewer calories over the course of the week. WOW! That equates to nearly the number of calories in a pound of fat!

Another excellent benefit of mint, aside from reining in appetite and helping to inhibit cravings, is that its fragrance produces a relaxing effect; it calms us. In a NASA-funded study, researchers found that during a stressful commute, subjects who smelled peppermint showed a 20-percent decrease in their levels of anxiety and fatigue and a 25-percent reduction in the intensity of their frustration. With regard to weight loss, increased cortisol levels from heightened stress can have negative consequences on your metabolic system—in a nutshell, anxiety can slow metabolism. The tranquil, soothing scent of mint can aid in the reduction of stress and keep your body functioning well. This detail is key, particularly for individuals who contend with "emotional eating."

Multiple studies have demonstrated that peppermint tea can also quiet the gastrointestinal tract and allow for healthy bowel movements. In short, it keeps the digestive process functioning properly. Mint can be useful in minimizing bloating and certain other intestinal problems as you journey toward weight loss and maintenance. According to the University of Maryland Medical Center, peppermint relaxes your stomach muscles and increases bile flow, thereby facilitating the digestion of fats.

I would be remiss if I didn't add two brief notes of caution: There is a chance that mint will interact with antacids, certain diabetes medications, and medications for other health conditions. Therefore, you should avoid ingesting mint if you have gastroesophageal reflux disease or a hiatal hernia. If you have been diagnosed with those illnesses, or you have any other concerns regarding mint consumption, please check with your physician. However, there's no reason why you can't enjoy the benefits of burning mint candles or lavishing in mint-scented hand creams, even if consuming mint isn't an option. You may even choose those other approaches if you happen not to like the taste of mint. My last caveat: I do NOT recommend the use of mint oil. In large quantities, it can be toxic.

Considering these facts and figures, why not try utilizing mint for its potential to further your weight reduction efforts? Take advantage of the hunger-suppressing and calming effects by burning mint-scented candles in your kitchen and dining room. Sip mint-flavored water or tea throughout the day. After meals, brush and floss your teeth with mint toothpaste or dental floss. I'll add that tooth brushing is a signal of sorts that your meal has ended, and you feel satiated. And chew sugarless, mint-flavored gum in between meals to quash cravings.

How does one wrap up a chapter chock full of tips? Perhaps the answer is to sum them up in one basic trick: **"Pick" mint and leverage the benefits of this versatile herb.** "Plant" it in your weight loss toolbox, and you'll end up—both literally and figuratively—in *mint condition*!

FOOD FOR THOUGHT... QUESTIONS & REFLECTIONS

1. Do you like the taste or smell of mint? In what forms do you currently enjoy mint?

   _____
   _____
   _____
   _____

2. In what ways have you noticed inhaling, ingesting, brushing with, or chewing mint has impacted your mood, eating behavior, or both?

   _____
   _____
   _____
   _____
   _____
   _____
   _____

ACTION STEPS & EXERCISES

1. Make a list of the type of mint products you might like to try incorporating into your daily routine. The choices are many; candles, body and hand lotions, bath oils, sugarless gum, tea, plants, and herbs for cooking.

    _____

    _____

    _____

    _____

    _____

2. Decide which items you would like to begin experimenting with and purchase them if you don't already have them on hand.

3. Over the next few weeks, start regularly incorporating one or several mint products into your life. Don't forget our other tip, "Out of sight, out of mind. In sight, in mind." Keep your minted items visible so you remember to use them.

4. Take notice of how each method of using mint impacts your mood and eating habits.

TIP #51

Experiment with yoga or meditation.

When coaching clients around weight loss, I always encourage exercise. In the past, however, yoga was not one of my typical recommendations, unless someone expressed a keen interest in it. Not that I deliberately discouraged yoga, but I wanted to impress upon my clients the vast benefits of increasing their daily caloric burn. I believed (possibly as many others did) that most forms of yoga don't provide nearly the extent of calorie-burning that aerobic exercise does.

I certainly never discussed meditation with those

clients either. As it was, the folks I work with need to find more time to grocery shop for healthy foods, cook more often, and go to the gym. Adding daily meditation to the "to-do" list didn't seem to make much sense if weight loss was the goal.

But today, I know better and, as such, must surely relay to you (as well as to current clients who are seeking weight reduction strategies) what I have learned. A substantial body of research has begun to indicate that both yoga and meditation can positively impact weight loss.

Instructors and personal trainers often share stories of clients who had lost substantial amounts of weight while practicing yoga. However, it is still difficult to determine whether or not the yoga in and of itself was the causal factor in their weight reduction. When I reviewed the data, I saw that several studies did, in fact, demonstrate that yoga participants experienced a decrease in pounds. Research findings were similar with regard to subjects who meditated and completed mindfulness training programs.

For example, in 2005, Dr. Alan Kristal of the Hutchinson Cancer Research Center led a trial involving 15,500 healthy, middle-aged men and women from which the data was subsequently analyzed. After teasing out concomitant factors that might also influence weight change—such as diet or other forms of exercise—the results verified that there was a connection between participating in yoga, shedding pounds, and sustaining the reduced weight.

Overweight individuals who began practicing yoga lost an average of five pounds, while subjects who did not practice yoga during the same period gained an average of 14 pounds. In spite of these statistics, from a scientific standpoint, it remained unclear as to how yoga might help foster and sustain weight loss. Dr. Kristal believed that the positive changes observed were related to the mind-body connection that is thought to be inherent in yoga practice.

The researchers suspected that the weight reduction effect had more to do with increased body awareness—specifically a sensitivity to hunger and satiety—than the physical activity of the yoga practice itself. A follow-up study four years later confirmed this hunch. The data from this experiment indicated that regular yoga practice is associated with mindful eating, and people who eat mindfully are less likely to become obese. Relative to his theory, it appears that yoga increases "mindfulness" and, thus, brings about a decrease in weight.

Mindfulness, particularly in its relationship to weight loss, has become a hot topic in and of itself! Mindfulness is the practice of deliberately paying attention to internal and external sensations in a non-judgmental, non-reactive fashion. The cultivation of mindfulness changes the relationship between our minds and bodies, and that can be applied to our perceptions of and, hence, behaviors regarding food and eating. Yoga forges a strong mind-body connection that yields wonderful benefits. One of those benefits seems to be a development in conscious awareness of what and how much we eat, sensing aroma, texture, taste, and satiation.

And that is why meditation comes into the weight loss picture. Meditation is just one of many ways to practice mindfulness. Becoming more mindful allows us to observe our bodies, our sensations, our thoughts and, accordingly, our actions. It follows, therefore, that through regular mindful meditation, we'll make healthier decisions around food choices. As a result of those decisions (electing to eat because we are physically hungry rather than as a consequence of our emotions or triggers from our environments), a shift occurs, and weight loss naturally follows.

A group of scientists at UC San Francisco conducted a study which established that meditation could be a causal factor in helping people control their dietary habits and assist them in their weight reduction efforts. The goal of the experiment was twofold: First, to employ mindful eating to help control cravings and over-consumption. Second, to utilize meditation as a means of stress relief and, in doing so, to prevent "comfort eating." The preliminary results evidenced that these theories appear to be accurate. The women in the control group gained weight while those in the meditation group maintained their weight and showed significant drops in their cortisol levels (high cortisol levels are a side effect of stress).

Dr. Catherine Kerr, a meditation researcher at Brown University, has been encouraged by the results of recent statistics, despite the fact that they were generated from a relatively small experiment. She stated that "These findings are consistent with numerous brain studies showing that this practice of attending mindfully to present moment experience brings about changes in brain areas responsible for body sensations, especially body sensations related to hunger and craving. A daily practice trains your brain to help you tune into your body in a more healthy way."

Aside from cultivating mindfulness, both yoga and meditation are known to be highly beneficial in reducing stress (as mentioned above). Nowadays, most people are aware that the more stress we experience, the more difficult it is to control appetite, emotional eating, and cravings. So any strategies or practices that relieve stress are excellent tools to place in your weight loss toolbox.

If you're intrigued (and I hope so, considering that you're referring to this guidebook to discover—and implement—weight loss strategies), why not integrate this approach into your new routine? With the advent of many specialty studios both for yoga and meditation practice, plus the explosion of classes in mindfulness techniques (usually called Mindfulness Based Stress Reduction or MBSR courses) held at locations worldwide, I'm sure you can find a class nearby. As the instructors say at the end of my favorite yoga class, "Until next time, Namaste."

FOOD FOR THOUGHT... QUESTIONS & REFLECTIONS

1. Thus far, what has been your experience with yoga, meditation, or mindfulness practice?

   _____
   _____
   _____
   _____
   _____

2. After reading Tip #51, what are your thoughts in terms of giving yoga or mindful meditation a chance to help you in your weight loss efforts?

   _____
   _____
   _____
   _____
   _____
   _____
   _____

ACTION STEPS & EXERCISES

1. Seek out and then sign up to for a yoga or meditation class this week. (Many studios will afford you the opportunity to attend on a trial basis.)

2. If you're shy or hesitant in any way, enlist the help of a buddy to take the class with you. (Remember Tips #28 and #46?)

3. If you're so inclined, read more about research findings of the mind-body connection, the relationships between yoga and meditation and weight reduction, or both fascinating topics. (See Appendix A.)

TIP #52

Respect your intuition and listen to your body.

I can hardly believe I'm about to introduce Tip #52! What an adventure this has been—one during which I hope you have acquired useful knowledge, incorporated these valuable tools and tactics and, most of all, have embarked on your quest to lose weight. Whether this was your first attempt at weight loss or your hundredth, this guidebook hopefully has encouraged, inspired, and assured you that weight reduction is possible without starvation, deprivation, or going on a diet.

Before I dive into this final tip, I want to congratulate you. Regardless of whether you have reached your "happy weight" or are still striving towards it, working your mind and body through this **weekly guide to permanent weight loss without going on a diet** is a true testament to your persistence and determination to **master the inner game of weight loss**. The fact that you've completed the entire guidebook is in and of itself an achievement worthy of note. So go ahead and pat yourself on the back; celebrate all that you've accomplished!

The final instruction, Tip #52, ties all components of this guidebook into what I hope is a beautiful, neat bow. I will share what I believe is the most important and relevant takeaway from this entire program. My wish is that you will internalize it as you go about your day-to-day life. Here it is, straightforward and concise: **Respect your intuition and listen to your body.**

So often, when people grapple with weight loss and maintenance, it's because they never wholly tuned into what their bodies are telling them. The human body communicates what it needs, what it wants, and how it feels. We just need to tap into our powers of awareness to "listen"—that is, to discern between real vs perceived signals.

We're all incredibly busy. Rather than well-thought-out actions, much of our behaviors are habitual. Especially in contemporary times, a good number of folks spend their days on "autopilot." Far too many individuals give in to mindless eating, immediate gratification, and convenience. Add to that all of the conflicting nutritional information that continually bombards us and it's no wonder the majority of people become confused.

Not a day goes by where there doesn't seem to be some

"new breakthrough" information touting the latest and greatest foods, drinks, supplements, diets, or exercise plans. All promise that, if we buy into what is being sold (pun intended), it will effect miracle weight loss or the fitness and vitality that has thus far eluded us. We're constantly being dictated the gospel—what to eat, what not to eat, and which diet and shape-up plans to follow.

However, we're all unique, and what works for one individual might not work for another. There is absolutely no perfect one-size-fits-all plan to follow that will lead to the optimal lifestyle and well-being for everyone. You must be your own detective and discover what works (and what doesn't work) to your benefit and what fits comfortably into your unique lifestyle. While that effectively sums up what I have intended to convey in this book, the fundamental message and method are not difficult: **You simply must pay attention.**

Having read this guidebook, you have learned to become cognizant of your actions as they relate to eating behaviors, the extent of your daily movement, your sleep patterns, your stress management skills, and your environment. I offer these 52 tips (and the suggestion to employ and reflect upon them) because all of the elements I just mentioned impact each other as well as your weight.

Now it's time to turn the reins over to you with this one last tip: **Tune into your intuition and the signals your body provides throughout the day and night.** After eating, ask yourself, "How do I feel?" Check in with yourself as to your physical and emotional sensations and overall perceptions. If you have fueled your body properly, you'll feel satisfied, energized, and comfortable in your own skin. If what you chose to consume has left you bloated, stuffed, gassy, uncomfortable, unfocused, and feeling guilty, it's clear that fare wasn't the best choice for you. This practice is this brief and this simple: *Begin to do more of what works for your body and mind, and less of what does not.*

Yes, simple, but not necessarily easy. Changing habits is challenging. However, it's not impossible. It necessitates a strong desire to act differently, and the belief that doing so will bring about further contentment throughout all aspects of your life. Trust that you have the power to modify your actions in order to become a healthier human being. These shifts and additions to your habits require practice and repetition. The more often you implement your new behaviors, acknowledge how much better you feel, and further approach your ultimate vision and goals, the easier it becomes to solidify new routines.

So off I send you, with the key to remember...The key that unlocks the door to new opportunities: **Pay attention. Tune in. Respect your intuition and listen to your body.** YOU KNOW what foods you should be eating to attain *and* maintain your target weight. YOU KNOW how much movement and sleep you need to function optimally. YOU KNOW how your environment, loved ones, and friends can influence your lifestyle habits for better or for worse. In the end, *you and only you* know what helps you feel awesome, vibrant, lean, and healthy. Just listen and follow.

Once again, I congratulate you and thank you for allowing me to guide you along this journey! You have successfully become a master at the inner game of weight loss.

FOOD FOR THOUGHT... QUESTIONS & REFLECTIONS

1. When you reflect back on all of the tips in this guidebook, which ones do you feel have become habits, i.e. behaviors that are now part and parcel of your lifestyle?

_____

_____

_____

_____

_____

_____

_____

_____

_____

_____

_____

_____

2. What tips have proven more difficult to incorporate into your daily life, that you also wish to practice further?

3. How often do you tune in and "listen" to your body and respect your intuition? What might increase your ability to pay attention to how you feel physically, mentally, emotionally, and spiritually, on a daily basis?

_____

_____

_____

_____

_____

_____

ACTION STEPS & EXERCISES

1. Pay attention.

2. Pay attention to your body.

3. Pay attention to the sensations and signals your body provides.

4. Pay attention to your intuition.

5. Pay attention to your thoughts.

6. Pay attention to your actions.

Thank You So Much!

I hope you enjoyed the guidebook as much as I loved writing it for you. I can't thank you enough for reading it and I hope to have the chance to serve you further at some point.

Although you've come to the end of this guidebook, you haven't come to the end of the journey. Continued weight loss and maintenance is an ongoing ride that takes many turns along the way. Whether you've reached your "happy weight range" or you're still striving towards it, it's important to continue building healthy lifestyle habits into your day.

So... If/when you feel yourself getting swayed by fad diets, gimmicky products, and false promises, simply refer back to this guidebook and keep practicing the tips and using the tools, because they will make your journey easier, healthier, and a lot more fun!

I would really love to hear your thoughts and feedback and any "AHA!" moments you may have had as you read through these powerful ideas, so feel free to send me an email at ellen@ellengcoaching.com and tell me what you think.

Be sure to join our Facebook group at www.facebook.com/EllenGCoaching, where you'll find daily tips, inspiration, and information to help you thrive both personally and professionally.

As an extra special bonus, I'd like to invite you to schedule a complimentary coaching call at meetme.so/EllenG so that we can strategize any potential roadblocks that inevitably will show up, and figure out your next best step toward continuing to build a healthy, thriving lifestyle.

To schedule your call, simply head over to www.ellengcoaching.com/weight-loss-coaching and sign up. I look forward to helping you in any way I can.

You can also feel free to reach out to me directly at ellen@ellengcoaching.com.

Thanks again, and I wish you great success as you continue to **master the inner game of weight loss**!

Ellen G. Goldman

ACKNOWLEDGMENTS

First, I have to give thanks to my many clients, both past and present, and subscribers who have been my lab assistants. Their willingness to try out many of the tips presented and report back their progress inspired me to write this guidebook. I hope it will end up in the hands of many others, and that there will be more and more individuals out there who will master the inner game of weight loss without going on a diet.

I recently received an email from a reader who followed my free program, *52 Tips, Tricks, and Tools to Permanent Weight Loss Without Going on a Diet*, upon which I based this guidebook. She stated, "***I did your 52 weeks program and have incorporated it into my life. I am down 25 pounds from last year this time.***" That is why I do what I do, and I have no doubt you too can have success by following my advice.

Next, special thanks to my friend Julie Lauton, who patiently and tirelessly read through every rewrite and gave excellent editing suggestions. She indeed is a wizard with words. Misha Gericke was a fantastic find, and she's responsible for the beautiful graphics, brilliant formatting, design layout, and final proofreading before we went to publishing. Andy Thompson, my business coach, marketing guru, and friend—without his constant advice and encouragement, this may not have come to fruition. Thank you all so very much.

Lastly, to my loving family and dear friends (you know who you are), who cheered me on and were kind and forgiving when I sometimes spent too many hours behind my computer rather than by their sides. It is their inspiration and support that propels me to continually pursue the best within me.

ABOUT THE AUTHOR

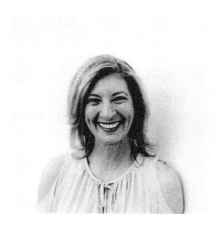

Ellen Goldman is a healthy lifestyle and wellness expert who has inspired, trained, coached, and presented to thousands of individuals throughout the country. She is a National Board Certified Health & Wellness Coach with over 30 years' experience in the wellness industry.

She created EllenG Coaching, LLC, to help overextended business professionals and entrepreneurs who are worried about their health and happiness, and who are either exhausted, burnt out, out of shape, overweight, or all of the above! She shows clients how to integrate health into their busy lifestyles with simple, small steps that lead to massive change, resulting in greater energy, focus, productivity, and happiness every day.

Ellen has been featured on the TV show, *Eye on New York*, and was a guest on several internet radio shows. Her articles have been published in periodicals such as the *Jewish News*, *Personal Fitness Professional*, the *American College of Sports Medicine Health & Fitness Journal*, *Identity Magazine*, and *Big, Bold Business Women of NJ*. She was selected to be the wellness expert author for *SparkPeople.com*, one of the largest diet and health related sites in the world.

Through her coaching programs, motivational talks, workshops and online educational programs, she shares her passion and the knowledge that, by building a foundation of health and well-being through ongoing self-care, you can thrive in both your personal and professional life. Ellen lives in New Jersey with her husband, Marc, and is enjoying watching her two daughters create independent, thriving lives of their own.

APPENDIX A

Resources

TIP #8

Bays MD, Jan Chozen. 2009. *Mindful Eating: A Guide to Rediscovering a Healthy and Joyful Relationship with Food*—Includes CD http://amzn.to/2yHKH7P

TIP #14

Wainsisk, Brian. 2007. *Mindless Eating*. New York:

Bantam Books. http://amzn.to/2zteMGv

Rolls, Barbara. 2011. *The Ultimate Volumetrics Diet*. New York: Harper Collins. http://amzn.to/2gIGzeo

TIP #19

Efficacy of water preloading before main meals as a strategy for weight loss in primary care patients with obesity: RCT. Obesity—A Research Journal. 2015 http://onlinelibrary.wiley.com/doi/10.1002/oby.21167/abstract

TIP #35

Sleep curtailment is accompanied by increased intake of calories from snacks. The American Journal of Clinical Nutrition. 2008 http://ajcn.nutrition.org/content/89/1/126.short

New study helps explain links between sleep loss and diabetes. UChicago Medicine. 2015 http://www.uchospitals.edu/news/2015/20150219-sleep.html

TIP #38

Eating attentively: a systematic review and meta-analysis of the effect of food intake, memory, and awareness on eating. American Journal of Clinical Nutrition. 2013 http://ajcn.nutrition.org/content/97/4/728.abstract

TIP #41

Wainsink, Brian. 2014. *Slim By Design: Mindless Eating Solutions for Everyday Life.* New York: Harper Collins. http://amzn.to/2zed0rI

TIPS #47-50

Professor's Study Finds That Peppermint and Cinnamon Lower Frustration and Increase Alertness in Drivers. Wheeling Jesuit University. 2017 http://www.wju.edu/about/adm_news_story.asp?iNewsID=1484

TIP #51

Regular yoga practice is associated with mindful eating. Fred Hutchinson Cancer Research Center. 2009. https://www.fredhutch.org/en/news/releases/2009/08/yoga.html

Effects of a mindfulness-based weight loss intervention in adults with obesity: A randomized clinical trial. Obesity—A Research Journal. 2016. http://onlinelibrary.wiley.com/doi/10.1002/oby.21396/abstract

APPENDIX B

Charts and Instructions

HOW TO CORRECTLY MEASURE YOUR WAIST CIRCUMFERENCE

A waist circumference greater than 35 inches (88 centimeters) in women or greater than 40 inches (102 cm) in men is associated with higher risk for type 2 diabetes, high cholesterol, high blood pressure, and heart disease. So knowing your waist circumference, and striving to lose enough weight to place you in a healthy range is important.

Here is how to correctly measure your waist circumference with a simple soft tape measure:

Take your measurement directly on your skin, not over clothing. Use your fingers to find the top of your hip bones. Your waist is the soft area and smallest indentation just above the hip bones and below the rib cage

Hold the end of the tape measure right at the navel and bring it around the front. Make sure it's not too tight and that it is straight, even at the back. Adjust it to the waist.

Take a deep breath in and then exhale. Check the number on the tape measure right after you exhale. Place one finger on the at the point where the zero end of the tape meets your waist measurement and read the number.

Repeat to ensure accuracy.

WEIGHT CHART

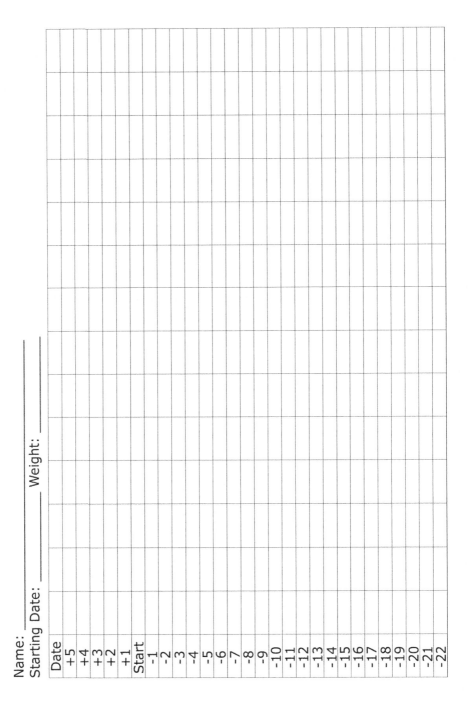

BMI CHART

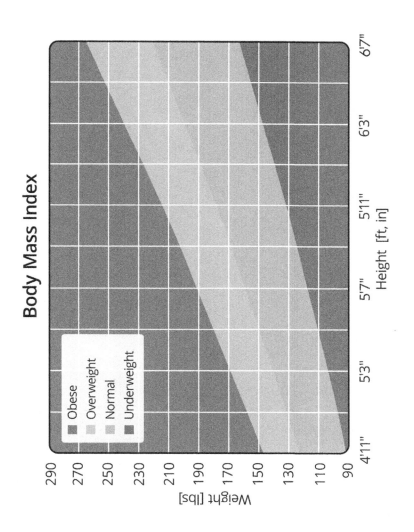

FOOD JOURNAL

Week of:

Food Journal

	Breakfast	Snack 1	Lunch	Snack 2	Dinner	Notes/Insights
Monday						
Time/Hunger						
Tuesday						
Time/Hunger						
Wednesday						
Time/Hunger						
Thursday						
Time/Hunger						
Friday						
Time/Hunger						

APPENDIX C

Suggested Products to Make Life Easy

PLANNERS

Full Focus Planner
Get 15% Off using the link below:
michaelhyatt.refr.cc/elleng

Best Planner Ever
bestplannerever.com?rfsn=429487.eb81e

TIP #11

Veggetti Spiral Vegetable Slicer
amzn.to/2yO8eFh

TIP #21

EatSmart Products Precision Calpal Digital Bathroom Scale
amzn.to/2xIWNtK

Salter Professional Mechanical Dial Scale
amzn.to/2wZ9e4U

Fitbit Aria WiFi Smart Scale
amzn.to/2xJ2qb5

TIP #31

Omron HJ325 Alvita Ultimate Pedometer
amzn.to/2xJFTQc

TIP #32

Digital Kitchen Scale by Zerla
amzn.to/2zcemDw

EatSmart Digital Nutrition Scale
amzn.to/2zei53A

OXO Good Grips Stainless Steel Food Scale
amzn.to/2wZ2Ev9

TIP #37

Zestkit 20 Pieces Glass Food Storage Containers Set
amzn.to/2x00ds8

Scotch Freezer Tape
amzn.to/2xICI6M

KitchenAid KSC6223SS 6-Qt. Slow Cooker
amzn.to/2xJBjl8

Ninja 3-in-1 Cooking System
amzn.to/2xKH5TG

The Complete Make-Ahead Cookbook
amzn.to/2wZ2Zya

TIP #42

Precise Portions—Weight Loss Portion Control Kit
amzn.to/2gU804u

APPENDIX D

Creating SMART Goals

As you go through the very many tips in this guidebook, some will be easier to implement than others. Occasionally, you might find that you are inspired to make changes, but doing so will require considerable attention and work. Examples of this might be regarding exercising more frequently or getting more sleep each night.

Breaking the behavior into incremental steps by creating SMART goals will increase your chances of success. Some of your endeavors are best achieved by setting a goal that will require small changes each week that will eventually have you consistently implementing the new habit within three months.

Below is an explanation of what SMART goals are and how to create them.

S = specific
M = measurable
A = action oriented (what it is you will be doing)
R = realistic
T = time frame

Three-month goals are the actions that will support you in achieving your long-term vision. (See examples below.) They should be written in the present tense, as if you're already doing the actions consistently.

Examples of three-month goals:

Fitness: I exercise five times a week doing activities I enjoy, for a minimum of thirty minutes. I keep track of my exercise sessions by marking them off on my daily calendar.

Nutrition: I eat a healthy breakfast every morning within one hour of awakening.

Sleep: I sleep seven to eight hours each night.

Weekly goals should be the smaller steps that you're ready, committed, and willing to take right now, which will support you in achieving your three-month goals.

Examples of weekly goals:

Fitness: On Thursday after work, and Saturday morning at 10:00 a.m., I walk the dog for thirty minutes.

Nutrition: On Thursday and Monday, I set my alarm for fifteen minutes earlier than usual, and eat a bowl of bran flakes and skim milk before leaving for work.

Sleep: This week, I'm going to bed by 11:45 p.m. Sunday through Thursday, rather than at 12:00 a.m.

RATING YOUR CONFIDENCE LEVEL TO SUCCESSFULLY COMPLETE YOUR GOAL

Once you've written a SMART goal, rate your confidence level for successfully completing that goal on a scale of 1–10.

1=Not at all confident.
10=Not a shred of doubt.

If your level is 6 or lower, ask yourself what would need to change, or what you would need to do, to increase your confidence to at least a 7 or higher. Sometimes, you might need to lower the bar a bit. For instance, rather than committing to exercise five times the following week at a confidence level of 5, perhaps making the goal three times a week would increase your confidence level to 8. Remember, you can always exceed your goal, but feeling successful is important! Or perhaps you need to rethink the times or days you commit to. You might need a Plan B. For example: If it rains on Monday, I'm going to walk on Tuesday instead.

Made in the USA
Monee, IL
31 January 2023

26802732R00197